Pain: Principl

practice and pati

D0245649

Beatrice Sofaer

THIRD EDITION

ıley Thornes (Publishers) Ltd

First published in 1998 by:
Stanley Thornes (Publishers) Ltd
Ellenborough House
Wellington Street
CHELTENHAM
GL50 1YW
United Kingdom

A catalogue record for this book is available from the British Library

ISBN 0-7487-3329-9

98 99 00 01 02 / 10 9 8 7 6 5 4 3 2 1

The cover photograph is by Andrew Lawson and shows *Papaver somniferum*, the
opium poppy.

Typeset by Northern Phototypesetting Co Ltd., Bolton
Printed and bound in Great Britain by TJ International, Padstow, Cornwall

Contents

Preface   ix

1   **Experiences of two patients who suffered unnecessary pain**   1
    Introduction   1

2   **Towards an understanding of pain**   11
    The influence of the arts   11
    Pain: a multiprofessional problem   13
    Ethical principles in the relief of pain   13
    Meeting the challenge of pain control   14
    Defining pain   15
    Placebo response   16
    Types of pain   16
    Patterns of behaviour   19
    Pain management programmes   21
    Problems faced by nurses in managing pain   22

3   **Psychological and cultural factors in the pain experience**   26
    Psychological factors   26
    The effect of learning on pain   32
    Cultural factors   33
    Psychological support of patients in pain by nurses   35

4   **Beliefs, responsibility, educational issues and communication**   39
    Beliefs and values   39
    Personal judgements   40
    Incongruence of beliefs and values within the team of health professionals   42
    Responses to and expectations of patients' behaviour   42
    Learning about pain relief   44
    Accountability versus power   44
    Partnership   45
    Communication   47

5 **Assessing pain**   52
   'Pain cues'   53
   Different responses to pain   54
   Difficulties in assessing pain   56
   Individualized assessment of pain   57
   Patients' views   63
   Prerequisites for nurses assessing pain   64

6 **'The cholecystectomy in bed 21'**   67
   Background and history   68
   'Clerking in'   69
   The admission   70
   The postoperative experience   71
   Home   73
   Pleasant feelings and pain   74
   Special people   74

7 **The science of pain: an update** – *Jackie Bentley*   76
   The gate control theory   76
   The physiology of pain   78
   Peripheral events in nociception   78
   Activities in the spinal cord   80
   Neurotransmitters   81
   Endogenous opioids   81
   The brain's response to pain   81

8 **Pain therapies**   84
   Distraction   85
   Imagery   86
   Relaxation techniques   88
   Analgesics   90
   Combination of pain relief measures   102
   Transcutaneous electric nerve stimulation   103
   Acupuncture analgesia   104
   Nerve blocks   105
   Other invasive procedures   105

9 **Feelings about pain and sympathetic listening**   108
   Feelings of patients   108
   Feelings of nursing staff   112
   One way of learning about feelings   113
   Despite scientific advances, people still suffer pain   115

Pain: 'a culture'   116
Nurses and nursing   116
Counselling   117
Concluding thoughts   120

Glossary   122

Further reading   124

Index   125

Foreword

We are living at the turn of the millennium, the age of high-tech. Everywhere you go you see things that only a few generations ago would have been considered little short of miraculous: microwave ovens, routine jet travel, colour pictures broadcast from the surface of Mars. Medical miracles are routine too: polio is gone, non-invasive imaging provides crystal clear pictures of your brain and heart transplants no longer make the headlines. So why is it that when it comes to pain, particularly chronic pain, we seem to be barely out of the Middle Ages?

Beatrice Sofaer paints a bleak landscape of the anguish and indignity that are the lot of all too many patients who have had the bad judgement of becoming injured or requiring surgery. How chilling to read in mid-book about Sofaer's own hospitalization. When it comes to pain even the shoemaker goes barefoot. Sofaer makes clear some of the relevant background. Too many healthcare professionals harbour undue fears of analgesic drugs. The result is underprescription by physicians, and incomplete filling of physician prescriptions by nursing staff. The well documented fact is that your mother will *not* become a drug addict because of analgesic treatment she receives in hospital. Another problem is the tendency to slip into 'ward routine'. Pain and its relief is a highly individual matter. Treatment following a rigid key is bound to leave many patients undertreated, and others perhaps overtreated. It is not certain why, but it turns out that it takes less medication to pre-empt pain than to get rid of it after it has already become intense. The aim should be to control pain before it has happened. Beneath it all, much of the callousness towards patients' pain seems to derive from persistence of the medieval attitude that, just as the sinner is supposed to suffer hellfire, patients are supposed to have pain. If patients and their families knew that a better standard of acute pain control is in fact available, I dare say that public demand would hasten its adoption. There is an important role here for education.

For Sofaer, compassion comes across as a special virtue of family, friends, nursing students and other medical outsiders frustrated for want of the tools and authority to 'really' help. Up the medical hierarchy people seem to become increasingly inured. There is undoubtedly some truth to this viewpoint, especially for acute pain. For chronic pain, however, the fact is that part of the reason we don't do better is that we don't know how. Both of the mainstay analgesic medications available today are old fashioned products from nature: NSAIDs are cogeners of an extract of willow tree bark (aspirin) and opiates are derivatives of poppy juice. Both drug families have severe liabilities for long-term use. There simply are no high-tech, low liability drugs for chronic pain. For many chronic pain conditions we don't understand where the pain comes from, or why there is so frequently a mismatch between the amount of tissue injury and the amount of pain felt. Serious research on pain biology is only just under way, and salvation through science still appears to be a long way off. So what is a soul to do in the meantime?

Fortunately, Beatrice Sofaer shines a beacon of hope onto this otherwise sad terrain. As she points out, we can easily learn to use the pain medications available in our armamentarium to better effect. But beyond that, it turns out that a special power to do good rests in the very hands of the erstwhile disempowered: family members, friends and junior nurses. That power is empathy. It lies in an awareness of the patient's pain, in the holding of a hand, in the restoration of dignity – in being there. Scientists have only a faint notion of how it is that a warm word can calm pain, but specific brain circuitry for 'endogenous' pain control clearly does exist. In the end, most pains are self-limiting and will fade in a few days or weeks. Just being there for your patients and your friends is often enough to imprint you in their minds as nurse-nurturer *par excellence*. What better satisfaction – and fully deserved.

Beatrice Sofaer is a passionate person with a passion for her subject. She has written a book for nurses, but really everyone should hear what she says. Ultimately, we all encounter pain, and would do well to know how to handle it.

Marshall Devor
Professor of Biology, Institute of Life Sciences,
Hebrew University of Jerusalem, Israel
1998

They were investigating one of the hummocky bits the Rat had spoken of, when suddenly the Mole tripped up and fell forward on his face with a squeal. 'O, my leg!' he cried. 'O, my poor shin!' and he sat up on the snow and nursed his leg in both his front paws.

'Poor old Mole!' said the Rat kindly. 'You don't seem to be having much luck to-day, do you? Let's have a look at the leg. Yes,' he went on, going down on his knees to look, 'You've cut your shin, sure enough. Wait till I get my handkerchief, and I'll tie it up for you.'

'I must have tripped over a hidden branch or a stump,' said the Mole miserably. 'O my! O my!'

'It's a very clean cut,' said the Rat, examining it again attentively. 'That was never done by a branch or a stump. Looks as if it was made by a sharp edge of something in metal. Funny!' He pondered a while, and examined the humps and slopes that surrounded them.

'Well never mind what done it,' said the Mole, forgetting his grammar in his pain. 'It hurts just the same, whatever done it.'

Kenneth Grahame
The Wind in the Willows (1946)

Preface

The first edition of this book was written in Jerusalem in 1984. I made an analogy then between the old and the new in that city and how much man had progressed in life and in the world of pain relief. The analogy is relevant now, but in a different way. Since then, one step forward and two backwards have been taken in an effort to make peace in the Middle East. In the journal *Pain*, Salmon and Manyande (1996) reported that patients who experienced bad pain and who were perceived by nurses as coping least well with pain were evaluated as unpopular and demanding. If there are nurses who still hold such unreasonable beliefs, then we too have taken one step forward in raising awareness by education and two steps backwards in not putting more effort into good practice. Despite advances in education, many people still suffer unnecessary pain. Health professionals have a moral and ethical responsibility to help them to manage it.

As in previous editions, I have attempted to introduce the reader to the concept of pain, but there are several changes and some new thoughts. There is the addition of an introduction to understanding the science of pain, contributed by my colleague Jackie Bentley, to whom I am very grateful. The sections on psychological and cultural factors associated with pain and its relief are updated. I have also included excerpts of narratives from patients on how they see the experience of pain and 'being in the health-care system' affecting their lives. In line with the rest of the book the chapter on therapies has been updated as much as is reasonable for a text of this size. I am grateful to Ms Sarah Grant, who is an acute pain nurse, for her advice on the relief of acute pain.

The book attempts to deal with principles rather than specific types of pain. This is because the management of pain (a complex subjective phenomenon) is a complicated management issue and is difficult. Understanding the principles will, I hope, lead you to ask questions about the specifics. Pain presents a challenge to health professionals and possibly more to nurses than others because we are in daily and continuous contact with people who suffer pain.

My own work in recent years has led me away from the wards and into a pain management unit where I have developed counselling within a multidisciplinary pain team. I owe a lot to my colleagues at Brighton Health Care NHS Trust and to the patients who have shared their experiences with us.

I have tried to make the text appealing to all grades of staff and to avoid complicated jargon. References have been updated, new research material has been included and a further reading list is provided. One could expand each section further because the literature has grown so much in recent years but there is a danger of the material becoming unmanageable and I want you to have a book that you will read (not just browse through). So, I have tried to encapsulate those ideas which I think will be of most use. I do also want to encourage you to explore other reading and to develop confidence in facing the challenge of helping people who suffer pain.

My thanks to my children, Joanna and Kirill Sofaer-Derevenski, Joshua and Esther Sofaer. They have a special place in my life in sharing love and affection and they help me to focus on things other than pain, such as archaeology, art and music! Louise Mestel has been a good friend since I came to East Sussex and I would like to say 'thank you' to her too. I am particularly grateful to Mrs Susan Bernhauser, Head of the Institute of Nursing and Midwifery at the University of Brighton. Her humour adds a sense of necessary 'insanity' to life and her friendship and support have meant a lot. Emeritus Professor Annie Altschul has remained a mentor and friend since my doctoral studies in Edinburgh and the first edition of this book. My colleague and research collaborator Janet Walker has made helpful suggestions for which I am grateful. All deficiencies in this book are entirely due to myself and not to her or anyone else who offered advice. My thanks also to Rosemary Morris, publishing consultant, for trying gentle persuasion!

There are many people in the International Association for the Study of Pain who have become friends and colleagues over the past 16 years. One especially, Professor Patrick Wall, has offered me so much encouragement in my studies, teaching and working with patients. 'There is,' he said in 1980 when I began, 'a life after a PhD.' What he didn't tell me was what that life was! Once you start to study pain it becomes a commitment, almost a love. I hope this book will encourage others to do likewise.

Finally, I am grateful to Professor Gabriel Josipovici for introducing me to the writings of Michel de Montaigne and for his permission to use the poem 'Unwelcome Guest' written by his late mother, Sacha Rabinovitch. Her poem speaks for many patients.

References

Salmon, P. and Manyande, A. (1996) Good patients cope with their pain: postoperative analgesia and nurses' perceptions of their patients' pain. *Pain*, **68**, 63–8.

Unwelcome Guest

Pain, that seasoned émigré,
has come unasked to stay.

Since courtesy forbids
probings and questionings

there is no way to know
when or if he will go.

By day he's on the prowl
seeking to gain control,

then creeps with clammy feet
by night between my sheets.

There at daggers drawn
we toss and turn till dawn,

for he will not retreat
nor I concede defeat.

Sacha Rabinovitch (1910–1996)

Rabinovitch, S. (1994) *Poems*,
Icon Bennett Booklets, Brighton.

For Carrol Siu, who did not ask why; but did.

Experiences of two patients who suffered unnecessary pain | 1

Every living being from its very moment of birth seeks pleasure, enjoying it as the ultimate good while rejecting pain as the ultimate adversity and, insofar as possible, doing his best to avoid it.

Racine

INTRODUCTION

Relieving pain, whether it be by providing general comfort or administering analgesic drugs, can be very satisfying. However, evidence from research and reports of patients' experiences strongly indicate that relief of pain is sometimes not achieved for a variety of reasons. The following pages provide some research and practice-based insights into pain and its management. In the final analysis, good management depends on the attitudes, compassion, skills and professional responsibility of those who care for people in pain. The aim of health professionals should be to maintain dignity and to support a person who may be afraid and worn down by the demoralizing effects of pain.

This chapter opens with two annotated accounts by patients of their hospital experiences. They do not make 'easy reading' but they are real, and give food for thought. The chapter concludes with some research material which is relevant to the experiences related by the patients.

The first section is composed of excerpts from an interview conducted in 1982 with a patient who underwent gastric surgery. The patient was a woman in her late 30s, married and with three children. The full interview appeared in previous editions of this book (Sofaer, 1984b, 1992).

Students of nursing are usually kind and sympathetic to patients but are so often caught in a difficult position. On one hand they are taught up-to-date attitudes towards relief of suffering, but on the other they do not have the power to actually sanction administration of analgesia or other invasive therapies. They frequently have to communicate with more experienced members of the nursing team who may or may not hold unnecessary beliefs or worries about addiction. The excerpt below is a good example of this kind of thing:

> After the first night I had constant difficulty in sleeping. The medication provided in my case didn't seem to work and I could find no comfortable position and, since the painkillers didn't work, nights were more or less spent sitting up in bed, changing to an armchair and generally wandering around the ward. The nurses (students) were very helpful but were, in most cases, unable to do anything since they had no authority to provide any alternative medication from that prescribed.

The patient had no real idea of what to expect. For her it was a unique experience, whereas for staff it was part of their routine.

> Had I not consulted my own doctor about the operation, I would never have been aware of what it entailed. When I had gone originally to the hospital, they had simply said 'an operation for duodenal ulcer'. I assumed it was being removed. It was my own doctor who explained that they were simply cutting the nerves which control the acidity in the stomach, otherwise I would never have known. On the evening before the operation a doctor did explain at that point, when I was already in hospital, what was being done but he gave no indication of how I would feel afterwards. I assumed I would have the operation, perhaps feel a bit sore for a couple of days and then all would be past. I was not prepared for the amount of pain that there would be afterwards, definitely not, and I would have liked to be prepared for that.
>   They [the nurses] took it very much for granted, perhaps because I wasn't nervous at all. I had no idea what it entailed and therefore wasn't nervous. I had no idea I could have taken so much pain or such a length of time, I really hadn't. Quite frankly I couldn't believe it was happening at the time. I felt it had to stop at some point.

The lack of effective pain relief was a total surprise to the patient but seems to have been taken for granted by the staff.

> It was very, very painful. The painkillers I was getting didn't seem to work. I don't know why but they didn't, they worked for everyone else. I assumed that sedation was so effective nowadays, it had never occurred to me that I would feel anything beyond twinges or slight aches, certainly not the throbbing and incessant pain that I had. It was 24 hours really. After the first 24 hours you are expected to sit up and put up with everything. I felt I was expected to. The pain relief that was available was not effective for me. They were willing to give tablets but they were no good to me. In fact, I think I felt worse. Everyone else seemed to find they worked. For me they certainly didn't. I did do my best to mention it to the nursing staff and in each case they said that this was what was prescribed, that the tablets were equally effective compared to the injection or

whatever it was I had been given before, and that the injection was too addictive. I wouldn't be allowed injections any more and this was the only alternative.

They said it wasn't time. I would be able to have something later. Eventually, they said, 'Right, we are going to give you an injection now', and I remember being turned over, given an injection and next thing I remember it was morning. But after that there were no more injections, I was simply offered two tablets.

There seem to have been fixed ideas as to when this patient was 'entitled' to intramuscular pain relief, yet she describes graphically how severe her pain was and how unresponsive it was to oral medication.

They didn't seem to believe that this could possibly happen. I caught the doctor at one point. I was utterly desperate and croaked to him because I couldn't speak properly, but I tried to make myself understood. I said that I had tried taking the tablets but they didn't work. I was having too much pain to put up with, could he please prescribe something that would help and he said, 'Oh, in that case we'll prescribe injections'. Well, when night-time came, and round came the medicine trolley, no injection had been prescribed and I was offered the same two tablets which I refused because they made me feel worse; and that was it really. It was a battle until more or less the last day when I had begun to feel that I could do without something. I just wanted to get home and try to take paracetamol or Disprin or something that would act as a painkiller and, in fact, I think I got more relief with Disprin than I did with the famous two tablets.

This experience changed the patient's perception of nurses and their role because of the way sisters (nurses in charge) related to her. She really was afraid of the possibility of future hospitalizations.

Sisters I found were totally unsympathetic. The student nurses at least were ready to listen and, in fact, I heard two say, 'You know, it's a shame when sedation has been prescribed, I don't see why it can't be given'. I remember that quite clearly at one point. Sisters, they had absolutely no idea of sitting down and listening – you would do this and you would do that and the pills must work – and no, absolutely no sympathy of any sort. They were very brisk. They seemed to see everything as a sick person's fantasy. I don't know – I found I got a lot more sympathy from the students, a lot more understanding from the students. They seemed to be able to relate better to your position than the sisters did. It was quite an eye-opener really, I now equate hospitals with pain, really, and before I thought they were fairly pleasant places, that they [the staff] were there to look after you. I must admit I have a different opinion now, totally.

I don't think I am particularly intolerant to pain and I am sure I can put up with it as well as the next person. It's just the fact that it was so unexpected and it lasted for so long. You almost felt like smashing your fist into something, simply to relieve the frustration of having to put up with this and not being able to get any help. I simply felt as if it was a nightmare and eventually I was going to have to waken up and find myself somewhere else. I remember thinking that quite clearly at one point.

Painkillers came only at particular times – at about two o'clock in the afternoon and then at night when the night staff came on. They were very fixed times, there was nothing in between.

The sense of frustration and lack of sympathy made a huge impression on this patient.

I asked once [for pain relief] after something had been done to the tubes in my stomach which brought on extra pain. I was more or less paralysed. I was finding it very difficult to walk and was told I would have to walk up and down, so I said, 'Could I have something to help?' and I got those two tablets after a lot of discussion with the sister on duty at the time. She said that moving the tubes shouldn't have caused any extra pain at all. I was having an awful lot of pain on one side which made it very difficult to move one leg and after a lot of discussion she seemed to go away and unlock something. She was unsympathetic. This is not the time to take painkillers. Painkillers were given at certain times. I certainly 'shouldn't have any need of them at this point in the day'.

It is obvious that there were priorities on the minds of the staff on this particular ward, other than that of relieving pain.

I don't think it [pain relief] comes very high on the list of priorities. It didn't seem to. There's a lot of care taken in washing and changing beds and keeping things clean. But no, pain didn't seem to be considered at all really. No one ever said, 'Are you in much discomfort, are you having any trouble?' – not really. There were exceptions, obviously, but on the whole, I'd have to say no.

The feeling of the unexpected happening on top of what the patient had already experienced added to her feelings of desperation.

The injections which had been given immediately after the operation seemed to be the only thing that really worked and there was only one that I remember being given. No, nothing seemed to work. Oh, another thing. I wish I had been told that I would suffer so much with wind after. I had no idea. I couldn't understand what these awful pains were creeping up my back until one of the other patients told me, 'Oh, this is normal, you get wind after you've had an operation, it's very painful and you have to break wind in some way or other.' I'd like to have known about that because no one thought to tell me I was having wind pain as well as, I presume, the usual aches and pains you have after an operation and I couldn't understand what this was. It was left to other patients who had already had operations and they said, 'Oh, these are wind pains and if you try walking and bending and taking drinks of hot water it ought to help to relieve the discomfort'. I would like to have been told that before. I'd have known what to expect.

It wasn't easy to communicate with people she had not known before the operation. The staff were complete strangers coming into her life at a time of crisis.

> When it was time to go home I felt I could talk to people because, I think it's the same anywhere, when we see a familiar face we tend to open up a bit more. At first, no, no, there was nobody I could really speak to. Because of losing my voice, I was at a disadvantage as well, because I didn't feel like speaking. I could whisper and they could hear but it was an effort talking and obviously I couldn't perhaps fight for things the way I might have if I had more of a voice and had it been less of an effort to speak.

Obviously she felt that this experience would affect her for some time, if not for the rest of her life.

> I think I now have a fear of hospitals which I certainly did not have in the first place. On previous occasions I found hospitals very happy and pleasant places to be in, really. No, I really would be very unsure of ever going in again unless everything is explained and I know exactly what is going to happen first and have been assured that afterwards there will be the minimum discomfort possible, but I certainly would not go in very readily. It would have to be more or less a question of life and death I think.

The experience of not being in charge of oneself and being totally dependent on others was very frightening for her.

> I didn't believe it was happening when it was happening. I really would have to talk to other people and find out if they felt the same way. I don't think they did. The other patients, they seemed to find, most of them, the painkillers were effective. I didn't, but people weren't prepared to believe it or accept that.
>
> One thing I could perhaps mention is the complete feeling of helplessness a patient has when in hospital. The layman simply doesn't realize what is going on. Doctors and nurses are so all-powerful and you are totally at their mercy while you are in. I remember lying there feeling that I had absolutely no power to do anything on my own. I was so totally dependent on doctors and nurses that I don't think perhaps they realize just how the patient sees them and how much in awe patients are likely to be of them. It's hard to explain. I think it may be fear, the fact that you are lying there and you cannot do anything for yourself. You know at any given time a doctor can order this or a nurse can say that and it will be done without you having any notion of why it's being done and what good it's going to do or how painful it's going to be. I think that's the main thing really, the fact that you are totally dependent on the nursing and medical staff or surgical staff whichever it may be.

Because she was ill, she was left with no option but to accept being controlled by others.

> Having gone through these various days of pain, it suddenly came home to me

that I really couldn't do anything but accept what was being done or not being done because I had no way of forcing my wishes on anyone or of explaining. I had to accept what was prescribed and what was said and all the rest of it.

[On being treated 'as a person'] Eventually. But while I was feeling very ill, no. [I was] a body in a bed that had to be given this and that. You were treated very much like a child in lots of ways. Sisters tend to talk down to a patient, definitely. Doctors are a bit better but the sisters talk down to you. Maybe it's the way I speak to my children sometimes when they ask for something which I feel is quite impossible, but I usually give them an explanation as to why it is quite impossible whereas in hospital you are simply told, 'No, that can't be done'. That's it, without any reasonable explanation of why it can't be done.

Feelings of hostility and resentment grew as a result of fear and anxiety about developing a complication.

After the operation you are expected to cough and bring up sputum. I have never been able to bring up sputum, I don't know why, even when I have a terrible cold I can't. But instead of being helped, I was told by sister that I would end up with pneumonia and a chest infection and, when I was lying there just longing for it all to be over, the thought of adding a chest infection and being in for so much longer was so depressing I could have burst into tears. It was left to the physiotherapist to reassure me that when my tubes had been taken out I would find it so much easier to cough and that there was no problem. I did not have to bring up sputum, I simply had to cough enough to move it around. According to the sister, I was heading for bronchopneumonia if I couldn't bring up sputum and I was very upset at that point because I felt I had another thing on top of the one I already had. Oh, it was horrifying. I could see days stretching ahead with me adding one illness on top of another without ever any way of improving the situation. So that was one point I remember, feeling very depressed one afternoon having been told this by sister, just two or three days after the operation. When the physiotherapist came she explained things so clearly that I realised it was nothing to get panicky about. But I had been told, 'You either bring up sputum or you end up with a chest infection, one or the other'. There was no choice and I was going mad trying to bring up sputum and just not succeeding. I actually got screens put round my bed one visiting hour so that I could continue trying without being in view of visitors and patients. Terrible, it was really frightening that. As it is you are feeling very low and very much in pain and the thought of getting some other kind of illness on top of it – oh.

You shouldn't menace someone who is already feeling down, it's no help at all. I'd say gentle encouragement, which is what physiotherapists tend to provide. They got an awful lot more results, definitely. You always feel weepy anyway when you can't eat and you can't do this and you can't do that, but to be threatened with another illness is certainly not the way to improve the matter. I remember feeling particularly resentful towards that particular sister ever after.

It is always a sobering experience to hear a patient's views. Several points brought out in the interview highlight the many myths about pain and lack of knowledge among nursing staff, in particular the lack of awareness about the individual nature of pain and the importance of believing a patient who says (s)he is in pain, together with the issues of accountability and communication in relation to nursing practice. The above account is one of tragic mismanagement of one individual's pain. Of course, this does not happen to every patient but, when it does, it can result in serious emotional difficulties, particularly if subsequent hospitalization is required. After the interview, the patient said, 'I'm glad I've got it off my chest. I can concentrate on getting well again now'.

The second and shorter excerpt is from a interview that took place in 1996 with a patient who suffers chronic pain.

Mr A sufferers from chronic pancreatitis. He is a family man in his 40s with two young boys. From time to time his condition worsens and requires him to be admitted to hospital. During the last couple of years his admissions have been a 'disaster', with staff not believing him and pain control being withheld or delayed. A plan was devised by the pain management unit, to supply Mr A with a letter signed by the consultant which would expedite admission and administration of analgesia when needed. He recalled his experiences graphically. He felt completely misunderstood and neglected by the staff and he put it down to their lack of education about pain management. But he knew how his pain would affect him:

> It wasn't very good actually at all, they didn't treat me too well because I think they haven't had enough training in pain and being a surgical ward they have a different philosophy. I became a nuisance. When the physicians couldn't do any more for me I became a nuisance and they wanted me to go as early as possible. One of the problems I found was with the medication; if I was on an infusion or injections those were always late and they could be up to two hours late before I got my medication. Of course I tried to explain to them that the pain would build up and I've had this illness long enough to know what it takes and when it's going to be worse than other times but I must admit it was like talking to a brick wall.

He began to get angry with the staff and was heading for confrontation:

> All the staff [behaved this way] including the doctors. But I mean everybody knows that surgeons have a different philosophy and I had a couple of run-ins with a couple of them. One didn't like the fact that I was on a pethidine infusion and patches and tried to take them away from me and I actually told him to go away and I told him the only person who was going to touch that was the doctor from the pain clinic and nobody else.

The staff didn't understand his pain. Following on from this he was asked what staff *ought* to know about chronic pain. He replied:

It's not tangible to them, [chronic pain] it's not like having an operation, having your appendix out or gall bladder when they've got a good idea how much pain you're in, but because I don't whinge and whine about it they think I'm okay and they think I shouldn't be there which isn't the case, of course.

Even though I had a letter from the doctor in the pain clinic, the attitude was the same because they do the obvious test, like my amylase, and because that was normal they automatically think that I shouldn't be there. That has happened in the past where they've asked me to leave and they wouldn't find me a bed. I was given a promise that if I had to come in again we would cut corners but even with a letter it didn't seem to register with them.

The effect of chronic pain on his life and that of his family was really very serious:

What they ought to understand, well, psychologically it can be very damaging over a short period and this is how I found it. I was at my lowest ebb when I was in there and they certainly didn't appreciate that, they don't appreciate what it's like to have pain every second of a day 24 hours a day, they have no idea and therefore you don't get much compassion whatsoever.

As regards my life, it's totally destroyed it. I mean I've lost a company, it's been a terrible strain on the children, for instance both of the children have been crying themselves to sleep at night saying 'We wish we had our Daddy back the way he was before' and my wife has a very demanding job as well and it's been a terrible strain on her. Tempers are short with each other, and then bursting into tears on many occasions. But we can't see any way out of this. It's something we have to live with and we've got to adapt to.

He was feeling very frustrated about the behaviour of staff and was asked to suggest ways in which we can help people to be more understanding of the kind of things he was talking about:

I don't know what I would have done without the pain clinic, to be honest. They've been excellent and at least they understand what I'm going through. It seems to me unless you're whinging and whining all the time people don't think you're ill and that's not my way. I try to fight it and then they think 'Oh, he can't be that bad,' I've been told 'you can't be in much pain if you're walking around' which is absolute total nonsense.

He went on to say:

... well, first of all talk to the patients involved so that they can tell them how they would like the people who are looking after them to approach them, to talk to them about it [the pain], to behave towards them, to try to understand.

He explained very well the kind of angry feelings he had when he was suffering:

Sometimes when you're in absolute chronic pain you can't always think logically and often you are in a bad mood and bad-tempered, which I would expect them to appreciate. But the first thing is they have to try and appreciate how it destroys your life, they must try and understand that. I've been ill now for three weeks and it was just sheer willpower that stopped me going to that hospital. I just didn't want to go there but in the end I had no willpower left and you know, I really really didn't want to go there but I didn't have a choice in the end.

The session ended with the patient's acceptance that he had now been heard.

I feel a lot better now I managed to get a little bit of sleep and I feel more comfortable now I'm here. I've got members of the pain clinic around me but unless I really have to I never want to go into that hospital again.

This excerpt is just one example of one problem faced by chronic pain sufferers – the pain of not being heard, of not being believed. It is not only a question of dealing with the world of health professionals. It is a matter of dealing with oneself, one's family, one's friends and colleagues. Having chronic pain means living in a world that is lonely, not understood and misperceived. It is a world to be avoided at all costs. It also means that negative emotions such as anger can be present. Fernandez and Turk (1995) explored the significance of anger in chronic pain patients and noted the consequences of anger for psychological and physical health.

There are some similarities between the experiences of the two patients whose stories you have just read. When nursing colleagues listened to the tape recordings of these interviews they expressed horror, embarrassment and discomfort. But most of them agreed that the experiences 'rang bells' and are by no means exceptional.

Research findings support some of the issues raised by the above experiences. Dodson (1985) suggested that attitudes of nursing and medical staff, the expression of pain by other patients, and the ward environment influence a person's response to pain. Sofaer (1984a) found that in a sample of 64 nurses interviewed, 75% admired patients with willpower and 80% held the view that patients sometimes exaggerate pain. Seers (1989) found that 43% of patients who had undergone elective abdominal surgery reported 'quite a lot of pain' or more on the first day after surgery. Twenty-two percent of patients rated their pain as 'very bad'. With regard to the fear of addiction, Cartwright (1985) found that 26% of nurses interviewed (n = 302) had reservations regarding opioid addiction and only 7% said they would give injections for as long as a patient required them.

Many difficulties encountered are to do with communication problems with health professionals. These will be discussed in Chapter 4.

References

Cartwright, P. D. (1985) Pain control after surgery: a survey of current practice. *Annals of the Royal College of Surgeons of England*, **67**, 13–16.

Dodson, M. E. (1985) *The Management of Postoperative Pain*, Edward Arnold, London, pp. 21–50.

Fernandez, E. and Turk, D. (1995) The scope and significance of anger in the experience of chronic pain. *Pain*, **61**, 165–75.

Seers, K. (1989) Patients' perception of acute pain, in *Directions in Nursing Research*, (eds) J. Wilson-Barnett and S. Robinson), Scutari Press, London, pp. 107–16.

Sofaer, B. (1984a) The effect of focused education for nursing teams on postoperative pain of patients. Unpublished PhD thesis, University of Edinburgh.

Sofaer, B. (1984b) *Pain: A Handbook for Nurses*, 1st edn, Harper and Row, London.

Sofaer, B. (1992) *Pain: A Handbook for Nurses*, 2nd edn, Chapman and Hall, London.

Towards an understanding of pain | 2

Pain forces even the innocent to lie.

Publilius Syrus

This chapter is intended as an introduction to understanding the concept of pain. It begins with a very brief perspective of pain as portrayed in the arts and then goes on to discuss the ethics of pain management. Definitions of pain are discussed and some issues faced in dealing with acute and chronic pain are explored. More attention is paid to the issue of chronic benign pain than acute pain. This is because its management is very complex and complicated and so merits more discussion than acute pain. Finally, some problems faced particularly by nurses in managing pain with patients are discussed.

THE INFLUENCE OF THE ARTS

Over time and in history we see that some ideas about pain have persisted while others have been modified. But generally there has been recognition that there is a relationship between pain and physical experiences which are harmful to the body. Pain has been written about both in prose and poetry and depicted in art and music from ancient to modern times. As Merskey (1980) noted, 'Understanding can only be brought about by experience and of all experiences that of pain and suffering is the most necessary'. He notes that writers may exaggerate but their ideas still 'have an appreciable force'.

Texts from Ancient Greece such as the *Iliad* and the *Odyssey* placed much emphasis on pain (Rey, 1995). Homer thought of pain as being caused by arrows shot by the gods. Plato argued that pain and pleasure were perceived in the heart and liver. Aristotle did not regard pain as a sensation but rather as a passion of the soul although he did recognize the importance of peripheral stimulation in causing pain. In the Bible, in both the Old and New Testaments, there are clear references to pain and to injury, for example in Lamentations 1:12, 'The Lord hath afflicted me'. In Isaiah 1:5, there is reference to pain in the body: 'The whole head is sick', and in 1:6, 'From the sole of the foot even unto the head there is no soundness in it: but wounds, and bruises, and putrifying sores: they have not been closed, neither bound up, neither mollified with ointment'. In Revelations 21:4 there is another example: '... and there shall be no more death, neither sorrow, nor crying, neither shall there be any more pain'.

In Milton's *Paradise Lost*, there is reference to pain. The following (lines 459–461) is frequently quoted:

> But pain is perfect misery, the worst
> Of evils, and excessive, overturns
> All patience.

It might be appropriate in the present context to think of replacing 'patience' with 'patients'. As was seen in Chapter 1, patients can indeed be overturned by excessive pain. It was an enormous relief when they had rest from it.

> For all the happiness mankind can gain
> Is not in pleasure, but in rest from pain.
>
> *The Indian Emperor*
John Dryden

C.S. Lewis, who died in 1963, is well known for his book *The Problem of Pain* written in 1940. A deeply Christian man, he wrote the following:

> All arguments in justification of suffering provoke bitter resentment against the author. You would like to know how I behave when I am experiencing pain, not writing books about it. You need not guess, for I will tell you; I am a coward. But what is that to the purpose? When I think of pain – of anxiety that gnaws like fire and loneliness that spreads out like a desert, and the heartbreaking routine of monotonous misery, or again of dull aches that blacken our whole landscape or sudden nauseating pains that knock a man's heart out at one blow, of pains that seem intolerable and then are suddenly increased, of infuriating scorpion-stinging pains that startle into maniacal movement a man who seemed half dead with his previous tortures – it 'quite o'ercrows my spirit'. If I knew any way of escape I would crawl through sewers to find it.

Art is also a powerful way to express and 'see' pain. The Dutch artist Van Gogh in 1889 painted 'Self portrait with a bandage'. He was a man who suffered much spiritually and is well known for depiction of his own suffering. Pictures by the Scandinavian painter Edvard Munch are often shown in lectures to demonstrate the visual effects of pain. He painted 'Despair' and 'Shriek' in 1893.

But nowhere is pain depicted more graphically than in the numerous pictures of the Crucifixion of Christ. The death of Christ on the cross is the central image in Christian art. How little or how much these images of pain and suffering influence people in pain is not known. It is a possibility, though, that in places where the suffering of Christ touches people and has an important meaning for them, their own pain and how they express it may be influenced by their religious feelings. It is not unknown to overhear a deeply religious person identify with the suffering of Jesus. 'He suffered for me so that I could be redeemed and now he is suffering with me.' (It is important, however, that a health professional does not expect someone to suffer because of this.)

Writers, poets and painters convey feelings about their pain or that of others. The French writer Montaigne wrote a lot about his pain in his essays (there are some more quotations in Chapter 6). He liked to quote the Greek philosophers and cited Plato:

> To be a true doctor would require that anyone who would practise as such should have recovered from all the illnesses which he claimed to cure and have gone through all the symptoms and conditions on which he would seek to give an opinion.

The same, of course, could be said of nurses and other health professionals.

PAIN: A MULTIPROFESSIONAL PROBLEM

Through the sciences as well as the arts, we know that pain is a subjective phenomenon. Many disciplines study pain. The International Association for the Study of Pain has members from a wide range of medical specialisms as well as neuroscience, psychology, nursing, and veterinary medicine. The problem of 'pain' is receiving more attention around the world because the answers have not yet been found. Researchers and health professionals alike recognize the issues and problems in providing relief. We know that pain can, when very intense, involve the total being of a person, affecting mood and intellectual ability. It is therefore important to believe a person who is suffering and to try and understand their behaviour and the meaning attached to the pain. This is a fundamental role which a nurse must undertake if she is to fulfil her commitment to caring.

ETHICAL PRINCIPLES IN THE RELIEF OF PAIN

It is questionable whether or not one should even think that the relief of pain is or could be 'an ethical issue'. There is a principle laid down by the International Council of Nurses (1973) which explicitly states that the fundamental responsibility of a nurse is to alleviate suffering. There are also principles which provide an umbrella for caring for people and central to these principles is the concept of respect for patients' rights. Sometimes the idea of respect for a person's rights may become obscured because of personal feelings held by a health professional. Thompson, Melia and Boyd (1988), in their excellent text *Nursing Ethics*, recognized that nurses, in common with the rest of humankind, may have 'perfectly natural feelings of like or dislike for particular patients'. It is very important that nurses recognize conflicting feelings and act professionally, that is, with a duty of care. The principle of justice is very important. Every patient has a right to proper medical and nursing care, physically and psychologically. We cannot evade or avoid facing the issue when a person is suffering pain and must consider what action has to be taken to relieve or control it. Basically, health professionals have two moral obligations to patients. The first is that there is a duty not to inflict additional pain and suffering beyond that which is necessary for effective diagnosis and secondly, there is a duty to do all we can to relieve pain and suffering (Edwards, 1984). Whiteway (1997), in her BSc dissertation, suggested that nurses do not always understand their ethical and professional obligations in relieving acute pain.

It may be useful to reflect on codes of ethics which, according to Tschudin (1986), describe goals and values which are important for the nursing profession. Throughout the world, codes of ethics reflect the respect that nurses should have for the dignity of patients, acceptance of cultural diversity and protection of patients from harm. It is questionable whether many nurses would think that pain control falls within their remit of 'being ethical'. One might argue that a health professional who fails to strive to control pain is not only acting without due professional judgement but is acting malevolently.

Because pain is an individual subjective experience, health professionals must be aware of the importance of believing a patient. Some health professionals still believe that they and not the patient should decide when pain exists. In so doing, one may amplify fears and anxieties. If health professionals feel uneasy about believing a patient's statement about pain, they are likely to fail in their moral duty since we do not have any objective evidence for the diagnosis and treatment of pain. We must rely solely on the patient to tell us what he feels and whether treatment is effective or ineffective. Somerville (1993) noted that one of the basic obligations of a health professional in relieving pain was that of developing trust with a patient.

MEETING THE CHALLENGE OF PAIN CONTROL

The contributions made by science, medicine and the behavioural sciences have improved understanding of the nature of pain and of the various treatments available for pain relief. For example, neurophysiologists have studied how the nervous system reacts to painful stimuli, pharmacologists have been interested in developing more effective analgesic drugs and psychologists have worked towards clarifying man's behaviour in relation to pain. Medical doctors have tried new therapies and nurses and other health professionals have become more understanding of their role in managing pain. Despite these efforts to meet the challenge of pain control, countless people still suffer unrelieved pain. Pain is the source of much misery in people's lives and the cause of much time spent off work. The number of working days lost through back pain problems for example was 60 million in 1990 (Waddell, 1992).

DEFINING PAIN

The perception of and response to pain are the results of complex interactions of many factors. For this reason there are difficulties in trying to define pain. People who care for patients in pain must appreciate that they are dealing with a wide range of biological and behavioural differences which it may not be possible to explain in any one way, since pain and injury are not necessarily related. The following definitions of pain point to its subjective nature.

Pain is a complex phenomenon, a signal of tissue damage threat, an integrated defence reaction and a private experience of hurt. (Sternbach, 1968)

Pain is an unpleasant sensory and emotional experience associated with actual or potential tissue damage or described in terms of such damage. (International Association for the Study of Pain Subcommittee on Taxonomy, 1979)

Recently there has been some discussion in the literature about definitions of pain, particularly in relation to those who are incapable of reporting pain themselves: newborn babies and infants, small children, verbally and mentally handicapped people and patients who are comatosed (Anand and Craig, 1996).

Because nurses have the most frequent contact with patients, an operational definition of pain may be helpful and appropriate. The following definition is adapted from McCaffery (1983): 'Pain is what the patient says it is and exists when he says it does'. (For assessment of pain with neonates and infants, please see *Further reading*, page 124.)

Wall (1977) went even further with his definition: 'Pain is'.

We cannot feel what the patient feels, yet it is not uncommon to overhear staff making comments that indicate they disbelieve a patient. It is important to recognize that every patient is different. A particular problem for patients suffering pain (notably chronic pain) is that the various specialists who see and treat patients have different perspectives of the same condition. The neurologist may talk of nerve pathways and the psychologist of the emotionality of the pain experience, each specialist perhaps not fully appreciating aspects of a patient's condition that do not fall within his own area of specialization.

Things are beginning to change though and as Finer (1982) noted, it is important that those who care for patients in pain have a multidisciplinary outlook. It is increasingly being recognized that a multidisciplinary approach to pain management is the most appropriate way to help patients. In the management of chronic pain, a programme which includes both medical and psychological strategies is most likely to meet a patient's overall needs (Waddell, 1992). This does not mean that nurses or other health professionals must be expert medical and behavioural scientists, but only that they should be aware of the complex nature of each patient's pain and of the fact that relief can only be effective if the treatment (or combination of treatments) is aimed at controlling all the factors involved.

PLACEBO RESPONSE

McCaffery (1983) defined placebo as 'any medical treatment that produces an effect in a patient because of its implicit or explicit therapeutic intent, and not because of its specific nature'. It is important to understand that because people are helped by placebos one should not imply that they do not suffer real acute or chronic pain, for no one can deny the reality of that pain. The placebo effect is thought to be due to suggestion, the wish to please the medical or nursing staff or the patient's belief that something is being done. Melzack and Wall (1996) noted that the greater the suggestion that pain will be relieved, the greater the relief obtained by the patient. In addition, they revealed that in certain circumstances placebos are more effective for severe pain than for mild pain. The area is controversial but it is likely that the placebo response would be more effective in the short rather than long term.

TYPES OF PAIN

Superficial, deep and referred pain

Superficial pain

Superficial pain involves the skin or mucous membranes. It is thought to be transmitted by rapidly conducting A fibres (see Chapter 7 for further details on the science of pain). It is perceived as distinct, short, well-defined pain and can be described as bright, pricking or burning. The nerve receptors of superficial (or cutaneous) pain are many and can be activated by various stimuli. These may be mechanical, electrical, chemical or thermal in nature.

Deep pain

Deep pain originating within the body is thought to be transmitted by thin, slow-conducting C fibres. This type of pain may not be well localized and usually has aching and diffuse qualities. Nerve receptors in the various organs are more widely spread than those of the skin. Stretching or tension may produce severe deep pain. In both superficial and deep pain, impulses are transmitted by pain fibres running in the sensory nerves to the posterior root ganglia of the spinal cord and from there to the cortex, where they are interpreted as painful.

Referred pain

The impulses of referred pain also travel to the cortex, where they are interpreted as painful, but pain is felt at a site other than that which has been stimulated. However, the stimulated site and that at which pain is felt are invariably supplied by the same or an adjacent nerve. For example, the fallopian tubes have referred pain in the shoulders and the appendix has referred pain in the region of the umbilicus.

Acute and chronic pain

There are several areas where health professionals have to face different problems in relation to pain management. Acute pain and chronic pain are different entities and although the same kinds of treatments may be used, they must be administered in an appropriate way because the management is different. Management also varies according to patients' individual requirements.

Acute pain

Acute pain has a sudden onset and a foreseeable end. It is accompanied by fight-or-flight features such as dilation of pupils of the eyes, increased sweating, pulse and respiration rate. Patients in acute pain are encountered in casualty departments, surgical wards and intensive care units. There are many techniques and drugs available for the relief of acute pain but, nevertheless, there is much room for improvement in their application. For example, postoperative pain is often suffered unnecessarily. This may be due to shortage of trained nursing staff. According to Scott and Hodson (1997), the general public has little knowledge about postoperative pain but high expectations of health professionals' ability to treat it. The Royal College of Surgeons of England and the College of Anaesthetists' *Report of the Working Party on Pain after Surgery* (1990) indicated that there had been little improvement since the first study of postoperative pain in the UK in 1952! A recent Working Party of the National Medical Advisory Committee in Scotland (Scottish Office Department of Health, 1996) published a report which recommended that traditional attitudes must be challenged and changed. Sofaer (1984) and later Davis (1988) both found a gap between practice as advocated in the literature and what actually happens. Thorn (1997) found that whilst nurses were aware of the importance of postoperative pain relief and its assessment, there were areas of negative attitudes, inadequate knowledge and misplaced beliefs in relation to postoperative pain control and its assessment.

Allied to the huge problem of lack of education and negative attitudes is the fact that the protocols for drawing up and administering intramuscular opioids are sometimes complicated and time consuming. Delays due to checking and administering opioids may result in patients experiencing unrelieved pain (Nayman, 1980). Sometimes delays can be avoided. Good practice means that pain relief is a priority. It has been suggested that the prescribing habits of doctors could be improved (Cartwright, 1985). The personality factors discussed in Chapter 3 may also add to the difficulties encountered. Furthermore, even if analgesics are prescribed to be given whenever necessary, patients may not be aware that pain relief is accessible. Even with the advent of patient-controlled analgesia, hailed as the ultimate answer to the relief of postoperative pain, there are still issues and problems to be dealt with. Hall and Bowden (1996) suggested that the introduction of a multidisciplinary acute pain service is the answer to the difficulties which continue to plague patients and staff alike.

Acute trauma

In a recent small study carried out as part of a BSc in Nursing Studies, Grant (1997) found that the attitudes of nurses working in accident and emergency departments were 'mixed' in relation to believing whether patients were suffering pain. Yet, there can be no doubt that one of the main reasons for attending A&E is because of pain (Selbst and Clark, 1990; Doverty, 1994). There is a special problem facing those who suffer acute trauma and those who encounter it in a caring capacity. The need for pain relief varies with the site of injury.

Comments from patients are useful to reflect upon. A fellow passenger on a train recounted to the author how he had suffered when having fluid aspirated from a very painful and swollen knee.

> It was outrageous. I never thought that pain could be so terrible. I had trusted the staff. They didn't offer me any painkillers either before or afterwards. I will think twice before allowing doctors or nurses near me again.

Chronic pain

Chronic pain is more of a 'situation', whereas acute pain can be regarded as an 'event' (Twycross, 1994; Richardson, 1997). Nurses encounter chronic pain, particularly in medical wards and during home care, more than other health professionals. Its management presents many, many problems, particularly because of the effect it has on the lifestyle of people who suffer it. It is important to distinguish between chronic pain of non-malignant origin and cancer pain.

Chronic pain of non-malignant origin may be accompanied by sleep disturbances, losses of appetite and libido, constipation, preoccupation with the illness, changes in personality and inability to work. The approach to managing chronic pain has to be flexible and should usually involve combinations of several treatments such as analgesics, transcutaneous electric nerve stimulation, acupuncture and psychological interventions such as relaxation therapy (see pain therapies, Chapter 8). It is important to realize that chronic pain from conditions such as sciatica, low back pain and postherpetic neuralgia is not life threatening, although the quality of a person's life is altered by having pain (Lipton, 1979). Pain frequently intrudes into a person's life to become the most important thing for them. The experience of pain destroys both personal bodily integrity and the presentation of a competent self (Kotarba, 1983). Kotarba describes three major stages in the chronic pain career. First, there is the onset, then the stage when treatments fail and then there is the patient's realization of the failure of medical interventions and the search for other kinds of help. This may happen over a period of several years. Finer (1982) describes the person in chronic pain as being 'in crisis' in that there is an inability to function psychologically as well as physically.

PATTERNS OF BEHAVIOUR

Working as a counsellor with patients in chronic pain over the last decade, I have found that 'crisis' frequently leads the patient to panic and that this becomes a habit through which smaller habits are formed. These habits become patterns of behaviour which patients describe as 'feeling low' (frequently labelled as depression), 'feeling worried' (frequently labelled as anxiety), 'sleeping poorly' (called 'sleep disturbance'), 'eating too much' (known as 'overweight'), misperceiving others and being 'mis-perceived' (called 'having poor relationships') and 'unable to manage time' (labelled as 'poor achiever'). As a result of these habits, the patient feels isolated, lonely, uncared for, unloved, frustrated and unheard. The following quotation from a patient exemplifies these feelings.

> I feel isolated and alone. My family and friends don't understand. We used to have such a lot of friends. They don't come to see us any more. My life has diminished. I no longer work. There is no quality to my life any more. It no longer exists. Nobody understands. Nobody listens.

The cause of these feelings is persistent chronic pain, the effect of which is that the patient, feeling so isolated, searches and searches for help, often seeking it from inappropriate or diverse sources. Sometimes patients seek help through a pain clinic, where they frequently describe having seen many doctors prior to the visit. The following story is typical.

> I have had pain for five years now in my back. I had been seeing an orthopaedic surgeon privately. He said he couldn't find anything wrong with me so I went to see a chiropractor my neighbour told me about. He said I had a problem with five of my discs. So I went to see another orthopaedic surgeon. He sent me to physiotherapy but that didn't do any good. My GP suggested I lose weight so I saw a dietician. But I didn't like her so I only went once. Then I spent a lot of money having acupuncture because my sister said that would be a good idea but that didn't do any good either. My GP doesn't know what to do. I tried some painkillers but they weren't very good 'cause they made me feel sick. I don't like injections – I will try anything!

Feelings of anger, confusion and frustration build up. Confidence is depleted and the patient becomes more fearful of pain. This results in a lack of trust in the medical and nursing profession and by the time the patient arrives in a pain clinic (or pain management unit) he or she is often surprised to find people who are interested and willing to listen. It is a relief to be able to begin to establish trust.

Having suffered for months or years in some instances, the patient may have developed what might be called 'immature behaviour', becoming demanding and egocentric within a family. One patient described how she went to the supermarket but only walked up the centre aisle leaning on a shopping trolley while her daughter rushed around the other aisles retrieving the groceries from the various shelves and returning to the centre aisle to place them in the trolley! This activity epitomized the patient's whole life where the rest of the family 'danced attention' around her. When this was pointed out to her, she then developed 'but' behaviour; that is, every time a suggestion was made which might help her to improve her quality of life, she interjected with a 'but'. She gradually began to realize that if things were to improve she had to take on more responsibility for herself and not rely on others. In a multidisciplinary environment she felt able to develop some trust. She began to use analgesics sensibly and worked out a programme of goals in collaboration with a trusted counsellor. These were aimed at reducing her fear, integrating her into society, developing good habits and being able to manage her time effectively.

Having done the rounds, so to speak, of the medical profession, she was unsure of her diagnosis. The difficulty in establishing a diagnosis was confirmed by the consultant in the pain management unit and the patient came to terms with this. She felt believed and heard. Then, in the knowledge that medical interventions might not be able to help her, she began to develop a little confidence in herself and to work towards achieving a balance in her life. It was a welcome surprise when she appeared in the pain management unit one afternoon to say 'thank you' for helping her 'to restore some balance' in her life. (The strategies used to help her were broadly those referred to in Chapter 9.)

What is required in many situations where people are trapped in the 'crisis' of chronic pain is an open discussion of the problems. Often fears can be dispelled by explaining to the patient that people who suffer chronic pain experience changes in their lives which produce negative feelings about all sorts of things and that this in turn may make them feel tense. Treatment will include the use of physical as well as psychological support.

Part of that treatment needs to be based on shared responsibility. The person in pain needs to relearn how to get back in touch with 'life'. A person suffering chronic pain frequently talks in the past – 'I used to (ski, run, garden, swim, play tennis or clean the house)'. The presence of pain has placed limitations on life and therefore one needs to learn how to prioritize. This means regaining control of one's life. The patient's body belongs to the patient and not to the doctors or nurses. A collaborative approach is required and this means patience, permission and persistence on all sides. The patient, for example, needs not to give up and the health professionals also need to recognize that they may become frustrated and bewildered by non-response. The issue of 'partnership' is addressed in Chapter 4.

Morris (1986) noted how, for the chronic pain patient, a night's sleep was so important and that some simple sensible measures can often help the patient to cope. Warm baths for example, can help relax tense muscles and not abandoning a sexual relationship can help too. 'Exotic positions may need to be avoided but a caring compromise is possible.' She also suggested that the back pain sufferer wears sensible shoes. It is surprising how often one sees back pain patients wearing shoes that throw out their posture completely. Health professionals should not assume that people will use their own common sense.

Non-opioid medications may be useful in reducing the level of pain. In general, care must be taken in the prescribing of opioid analgesic drugs as some patients may develop dependence. However, in some very severe and intractable situations, they are used successfully.

An important aspect to consider when dealing with patients suffering chronic pain of non-malignant origin, is the process of adaptation. Somehow, some individuals may manage to endure pain and carry on despite it. They may appear untroubled and may get through their work by means of sheer willpower, although there may be accompanying signs of depression. Staff may then, erroneously, be more concerned with the apparent depression than with the underlying unexpressed pain which is its cause. Walker *et al.* (1989) suggested that when pain cannot be cured or eliminated, as is often the case with sufferers of chronic pain, the patient must learn to cope with or gain control over the pain and in so doing may need help. Patients sometimes report that their pain is influenced by changes in the weather (Jamison, Anderson and Slater, 1995). Cold and damp weather seems to affect chronic pain the most. Patients may need help to develop coping strategies to deal with this problem (see Chapter 3).

One patient who sustained a serious back injury when he fell off a ladder described how he was trying to cope and adapt 'normally'. He said:

> I have no feeling in one leg but I try to carry on my life normally. My back hurts like hell sometimes. I have to be realistic. I am carrying on my business. I'm not going to let that go down the drain after 12 years. I know I can't go away with the lads next weekend but I have some plans to keep me occupied.

Counselling helped him to establish realistic goals and to learn to appreciate what he was able to do successfully. But he maintained (and he was probably correct) that being disabled halfway through life was a great deal harder than having to cope with it from birth.

PAIN MANAGEMENT PROGRAMMES

A pain management programme is a rehabilitative treatment programme which is psychologically based and geared toward people with chronic pain who have not responded to available medical and other physical treatments. The aim of such a programme is to reduce the distress and disability of pain sufferers by teaching them psychological, physical and practical measures to improve the quality of their life. Pain relief may not be the first priority but teaching patients to be as reliant on themselves as possible is. The Pain Society (the British and Irish Chapter of the International Association for the Study of Pain) recently published a *Report of a Working Party on Desirable Criteria for Pain Management Programmes* (Pain Society, 1996). These guidelines included issues to do with referral and selection of patients as well as the inclusion of key clinical multidisciplinary staff.

Sickle cell disease pain

Painful crises are frequently experienced by people who suffer from sickle cell disease, a hereditary disease which affects Caribbean and African people. Although the same principles of management apply to any person suffering pain, according to Thomas (1997) in an excellent chapter about pain management in this group of people, it appears to be a particular problem. The reader is urged to consult Thomas for further information about the disease and its pain management.

Cancer pain

Cancer pain is managed differently from chronic pain of non-malignant origin. There is a need for carers to be aware that open communication between nurses, patients and doctors will be of help to patients in living their last days free from fear and anxiety. With cancer, one is dealing with a process of progressive change. It is important to review pain relief regularly because the pattern of pain may change. All aspects of body and mind comfort should be attended to. With cancer pain, patients may have both the fight-or-flight reactions normally associated with acute pain as well as insomnia, lack of appetite and loss of libido, constipation, personality changes, preoccupation with symptoms and lack of interest in work. If cancer pain is not controlled, patients become very demoralized and wearied by suffering. Good management of cancer pain seeks to support the cancer patient by the provision of adequate medication, comfort, rest and attention. The relief of pain and symptoms in the management of cancer is a very large topic and it is strongly suggested that the reader consults a specialist text on the subject, such as Twycross (1994) and Richardson (1997).

   Wherever a nurse or other health professional is caring for a patient in pain, be it in areas of acute care or in the management of chronic or terminal pain, it is important to be constantly aware that judgemental attitudes, disbelief and withholding pain relief are not helpful when 'it hurts'.

PROBLEMS FACED BY NURSES IN MANAGING PAIN

When asked about problems they faced in trying to help patients in pain, groups of nurses identified the following difficulties:

For patients with acute pain

- Lack of awareness among nursing staff of severity of patients' pain.
- Fear among nurses of masking symptoms by analgesia.
- Acceptance of analgesia regime without seeking alternatives.
- Lack of recording of patients' pain.
- Ignorance of drug efficacies.
- Problems of communication between nurses, patients and doctors.

For patients with chronic pain

- Referrals to several different specialists or doctors resulting in patients being given different and sometimes conflicting explanations and/or information.
- Coping with patients' depression, anxiety and hostility in general wards.
- Helping patients to cope with life.
- Physical manifestations of pain may not be present.
- Frustration among staff.
- Problems of communication between patients and staff.
- Lack of knowledge about therapies.
- Lack of knowledge about the nature of chronic pain.

For patients terminally ill at home

- Helping the patient to cope.
- Educating relatives and helping them to cope.
- Communication between nursing staff and the general practitioner.
- Difficulties of liaison with hospital.
- Lack of knowledge about therapies.

For patients terminally ill in hospital

- Lack of privacy for the patient.
- Ignorance among staff regarding pain control.
- Problems of communication between patients, relatives, nurses and doctors.

It is not within the scope of this book to cover all the points mentioned above. However, nurses' awareness that these problems exist and that they are serious issues will go some way towards facing the challenge of pain control.

References

Anand, K. J. S. and Craig, K. D. (1996) New perspectives on the definition of Pain. *Pain*, **67**(1), 3–6.

Cartwright, P. D. (1985) Pain control after surgery: a survey of current practice. *Annals of the Royal College of Surgeons of England*, **67**, 13–16.

Davis, P. S. (1988) Changing nursing practice for more effective control of post-operative pain through a staff initiated educational programme. *Nurse Education Today*, **8**, 325–31.

Doverty, N. (1994) Make pain assessment your priority. Practitioner-led management of pain in trauma injuries. *Professional Nurse*, January, 230–7.

Edwards, R. B. (1984) Pain and the ethics of pain management. *Social Science and Medicine*, **18**, 515–23.

Finer, B. (1982) Treatment in an interdisciplinary pain clinic, in *Psychological Approaches to the Management of Pain*, (eds J. Barber and C. Adrian), Brunner Mazel, New York.

Grant, S. (1997) Staff perceptions of pain management in accident and emergency departments. Unpublished BSc dissertation. University of Brighton.

Hall, P. A. and Bowden, M. I. (1996) Introducing an acute pain service. *British Journal of Hospital Medicine*, **55** (1/2), 15–17.

International Association for the Study of Pain Subcommittee on Taxonomy (1979) Pain terms: a list with definitions and notes on usage. *Pain*, **6**, 249–52.

International Council of Nurses (1973) *Code for Nurses: Ethical Concepts Applied to Nursing*, International Council of Nurses, Geneva.

Jamison, R. N., Anderson, K. O. and Slater, M. A. (1995) Weather changes and pain: perceived influence of local climate on pain complaint in chronic pain. *Pain*, **61**(2), 309–15.

Kotarba, J. A. (1983) *Chronic Pain. Its Social Dimensions*, Sage Publications, Beverly Hills.

Lewis, C. S. (1940) *The Problem of Pain*, Century Press, London.

Lipton, S. (1979) The treatment of chronic pain, in *The Control of Chronic Pain*, (ed. S. Lipton), Edward Arnold, London.

McCaffery, M. (1983) *Nursing the Patient in Pain*, Harper and Row, London.

Melzack, R. and Wall, P. D. (1996) *The Challenge of Pain*, Penguin Books, Harmondsworth.

Merskey, H. (1980) Some features of the history of pain. *Pain*, **9**, 3–8.

Morris, R. (1986) Life goes on with chronic pain. A personal account. *Nursing*, **10**, 375–6.

Nayman, J. (1980) Control of postoperative pain: a multidisciplinary approach, in *Proceedings of the First Australia-New Zealand Conference on Pain*, (eds C. Peck and M. Wallace), Pergamon Press, Oxford.

Pain Society (1996) Desirable criteria for pain management programmes. Report of a Working Party of the Pain Society, 1995. *Journal of the Pain Society*, 12, 12–15.

Rey, R (1995) *History of Pain*, Harvard University Press, Cambridge, Mass.

Richardson, A. (1997) Cancer pain and its management, in *Pain. Its Nature and Management*, (ed. V. N. Thomas), Baillière Tindall, London.

Royal College of Surgeons of England and the College of Anaesthetists (1990) *Report of the Working Party on Pain After Surgery*, Royal College of Surgeons of England and the College of Anaesthetists, London.

Scott, N. B. and Hodson, M. (1997) Public perceptions of postoperative pain and its relief. *Anaesthesia*, **52**, 438–42.

Scottish Office Department of Health (1996) *Provision of Services for Acute Post-operative Pain in Scotland, A Report by the National Medical Advisory Committee*, HMSO, Edinburgh.

Selbst, M. and Clark, M. (1990) Analgesic use in the Emergency Department. *Annals of Emergency Medicine*, **19**(9), 99–102.

Sofaer, B. (1984) The effect of focused education for nursing teams on post-operative pain of patients. Unpublished PhD thesis, University of Edinburgh.

Somerville, M. A. (1993) Pain, suffering and ethics. *Paper presented to the 7th World Congress on Pain*, Paris.

Sternbach, R. A. (1968) *Pain: A Psychophysiological Analysis*, Academic Press, New York.

Thomas, V. N. (1997) Sickle cell disease pain, in *Pain. Its Nature and Management*, (ed. V. N. Thomas), Baillière Tindall, London.

Thompson, I. E. Melia, K. M. and Boyd, K. M. (1988) *Nursing Ethics*, Churchill Livingstone, Edinburgh.

Thorn, M. (1997) A survey of nurses' attitudes towards the assessment and control of postoperative pain. *Journal of Orthopaedic Nursing*, **1**(11), 30–8.

Tschudin, V. (1986) *Ethics in Nursing – The Caring Relationship*, Heinemann Nursing, London.

Twycross, R. G. (1994) *Pain Relief in Far Advanced Cancer*, Churchill Livingstone, Edinburgh.

Waddell, G. (1992) Biopsychosocial analysis of low back pain. *Baillière's Clinical Rheumatology*, **6**, 523–57.

Walker, J. M., Akinsanya, J. A., Davis, B. D. and Marcer, D. (1989) The nursing management of pain in the community: a theoretical framework. *Journal of Advanced Nursing*, **14**, 247.

Wall, P. D. (1977) Why do we not understand pain?, in *The Encyclopaedia of Ignorance*, (eds. R. Duncan and M. Weston-Smith), Pergamon Press, Oxford, 361–8.

Whiteway, S.A. (1997) What are the factors influencing clinical decision making in acute pain management for patients prescribed intramuscular analgesia? Unpublished BSc dissertation, University of Brighton.

3

Psychological and cultural factors in the pain experience

> The evidence shows that pain is much more variable and modifiable than many people have believed in the past. Pain differs from person to person, culture to culture.
>
> *Melzack and Wall, 1996*

This chapter addresses some of the psychological and cultural factors that are important to consider in pain management. Quotations from a patient who suffered 47 years of phantom leg pain will illustrate the concept of individuality. Some 'older' references from previous editions of this book have been retained because of their importance in contributing to the understanding of psychological and cultural factors in the experience of pain.

PSYCHOLOGICAL FACTORS

There is no predictable relationship between pain and injury. Each individual's pain experience is influenced by his unique personal history, by the meaning he attaches to his pain and by his state of mind. People with the same or similar conditions will behave differently because of variations in background and personality. It is important for health professionals, and particularly nurses, to recognize this and to realize the crucial part that psychology plays in behaviour during illness.

Many health carers think that they, not the patient, can decide how intense pain is. Taylor, Skelton and Butcher (1983), in a study of hypothetical patients, found that nurses attributed less pain to patients who displayed no obvious signs of suffering.

Sometimes patients adapt to pain both physiologically and behaviourally so that it is not easy for carers to see if a patient is suffering. Minimal expressions of pain may therefore be misunderstood. Sometimes the cause of pain may not be easy to identify and a patient's pain may be erroneously dismissed by staff. But we must accept that all pain is real, regardless of its cause, and that most bodily pain probably results from a combination of physical and psychological factors.

A knowledge of psychological factors associated with pain will be helpful in understanding patients' reactions. Pain perception however is not a simple concept. Areas of psychology that are particularly relevant are the relationship of anxiety, depression and anger to pain. A range of negative emotions may accompany either acute or chronic pain but anxiety is particularly associated with acute pain. Anxiety, depression and anger may be present in chronic pain.

Emotions, moods and beliefs

It would seem reasonable to expect that heightened emotions, i.e. being anxious, depressed or angry, would influence one's perception of pain (Vingoe, 1994). But as Wade et al. (1990) have noted, pain is a multidimensional problem.

The concept of 'coping' is discussed below but in relation to emotion, it is worth noting that beliefs about 'control' are related to coping. A study of patients suffering chronic pain carried out by Crisson and Keefe (1988) confirmed that patients with strong beliefs that their health was controlled by chance were more likely to be depressed, anxious and obsessive, and to experience greater distress than patients with weaker beliefs.

What people believe about their pain may have important implications for the way it is managed. Skevington (1995) noted that greater success in treatment may be achieved by matching the style of treatment to a person's beliefs, unless the treatment is aimed at changing beliefs. Skevington also pointed out that the environment and social context in which a patient finds himself are important in influencing his reaction to pain. Craig and Best (1977) reported that pain perception is also affected by the way other people around the patient react to pain. People also have differing expectations about the amount and kind of pain relief which will be made available to them. Carr (1997) noted that on the whole the expectations of the public are low and it is probably because of this that there has not been public outrage about inadequate pain management.

Pain is often regarded merely as a symptom of physical or mental illness. It is important that pain is dealt with from both the physical and the psychological standpoints.

The influence of personality on people's pain tolerance and pain thresholds has been studied by many researchers. In general, pain thresholds have been found to be lower for introverted people than for extroverts, but extroverts have tended to report pain more freely. In one early study, it was found that extrovert subjects received more analgesia than introvert subjects (Bond and Pearson 1969). In terms of emotionality, those who are most emotional may have the most pain (Bond, 1979). Research in the 1980s and 1990s has concentrated more on individual coping styles than on personality types.

It may be helpful to both staff and patients for a nurse to ask each patient on admission how he sees himself in terms of coping. It can be useful for staff to have a record on the care plan of how each patient usually reacts to illness and stress and his attitude to a particular admission to hospital. It is helpful for a patient to know that staff are aware of how he normally copes with pain. It should also be made clear to patients at this time what provisions will be made for pain relief. Staff take it for granted that they will provide some sort of analgesia, but patients like to know. If nothing else, it lets the patient know that staff are interested in him as a person and in his well-being, before, during and after a potentially painful event. This knowledge alone may have a pronounced effect in reducing anxiety, particularly in over-anxious people whose apprehension may be based, among other things, on the fear of pain itself.

Depression

Some people respond to stress by feeling a little low, while others feel a sense of despair. Patients in pain, particularly those who experience chronic pain and have had their lives altered by their inability to function socially or perform activities of daily living, may experience considerable depression. Obviously, if a person normally has a tendency to feel low he will be more likely to suffer despair as a result of chronic pain. Coping with pain becomes even more difficult in these circumstances. It is important for nurses to be aware of these factors when supporting patients. Assessment of depression, however, is difficult in patients who suffer chronic pain because there is an overlap of symptoms between the two (Romano and Turner, 1985). The reader is referred to an excellent book on the psychology of pain by Skevington (1995), in which she discusses the literature on the relationship between depression controllability, attributions and cognitive distortions. She highlights the notion of 'learned helplessness' in which some people become used to thinking about events in such a way that they become helpless and depressed when faced with unpleasant events. Central to this idea is the notion that 'helpless' people have lost control over unpleasant events which happen in their lives.

Anxiety

Most people become apprehensive when faced with a painful illness. Those who tend to be worriers by nature, when confronted by such an event, may become so anxious that they are overwhelmed. For these patients, pain may be greater because pain causes anxiety (particularly acute pain) and anxiety, in turn, may heighten pain perception. On the other hand, pain may precede anxiety or depression (Casten *et al.*, 1995).

It has been reported that preparing a patient in advance for surgery by giving information and teaching coping techniques may help (Johnson, Dabbs and Leventhall, 1970). In addition, research by Hayward (1975), Boore (1977) and Davis (1988) has shown that in terms of anxiety reduction and consequent decreased postoperative pain, it may benefit patients to have preoperative information. Fear of the unknown may compound the pain experience. The patient in pain may have lost self-esteem; information may give them insight. The underlying idea is that, if a person can understand better what to expect, this understanding will reduce his anxiety and, in turn, his pain. However, it is important to know something about the patient's feelings in relation to his normal anxiety level. A moderately anxious person may do a little 'worry work' which can be helpful in building up psychological defences to deal with the stress, but those whose normal anxiety level is either very high or very low may be at a disadvantage. This was demonstrated by Janis (1958) in his seminal work. Jensen, Karoly and Harris (1991) examined how both anxiety and depression affected adjustment in chronic pain patients.

Anger

Although many studies have confirmed that depression and anxiety are important concomitants of chronic pain, evidence is emerging that anger is also an important component of chronic pain experience. Wade *et al.* (1990) suggested that anger and frustration are important components of the emotional unpleasantness suffered by people with chronic pain. Fernandez and Turk (1995) reviewed the scope and significance of anger in the experience of chronic pain. They concluded that the prevalence of anger among chronic pain patients should be seen as important because it can have 'deleterious consequences' for the physical and psychosocial well-being of patients. Anger may be particularly strong if the damage was a result of something which was avoidable or preventable. Health professionals find it very difficult to deal with anger.

Coping

Traditionally, the concept of coping has been associated with focusing on strategies to do with emotions and problems (Folkman and Lazarus, 1980). Jensen *et al.* (1991) reviewed the literature on coping and suggested that patients who believe that they can control their pain and that they are not severely disabled appear to function better than patients who don't hold those beliefs. Brown and Nicassio (1987) had earlier developed a measure of coping, the Vanderbilt Pain Management Inventory (VPMI), which classified active versus passive coping strategies. They defined active coping strategies as those which chronic pain sufferers use when attempting to control their pain and/or to maintain functioning despite its presence, whereas passive coping strategies are those where patients allow others to control the pain or allow areas in their life to be affected by the pain.

Snow-Turek, Norris and Tan (1996) note that these definitions were expanded on by Nichols, Wilson and Goyen (1992) who specified that 'active strategies involve an attempt by the patient to use his/her resources, and passive strategies are characterized by helplessness and/or reliance on others'. Snow-Turek, Norris and Tan (1996) developed the idea of active versus passive coping further and using the Coping Strategies Questionnaire (developed by Rosenstiel and Keefe in 1983), they found that passive coping strategies were associated with 'maladaptive physical and psychological functioning' and active coping strategies were associated with 'greater physical activity and decreased maladaptive psychological functioning'. Although the findings were from a sample of patients who were very physically and psychologically impaired, it is worth noting the kind of items that classified them into either active or passive copers; for example, the 'active copers' reported constructs like 'not thinking about the pain', 'thinking of something pleasant', 'thinking of another sensation such as numbness', 'keeping going', 'pretending it is not part of me'. 'Passive copers' on the other hand, reported constructs such as 'it overwhelms me', 'I pray God it won't last long', 'I have faith in doctors that someday there will be a cure for my pain' and 'can't stand it any more'.

People do vary very much and an over-anxious individual may find difficulty in developing the inner strength to cope, whereas a very calm person may be quite disagreeably surprised by the inescapable stress and pain. Differences in coping styles are understandable since different past experiences, variations in availability of resources and in social and family support affect individuals in different ways. Coping may vary from day to day. Keefe *et al.* (1997) described a study where patients who had rheumatoid arthritis kept a daily diary of coping strategies and coping efficacy that occurred during treatment of their condition. Reviewing the diary was helpful to patients. The findings of the study suggested that patients who cope less well during a period of bad pain may be at risk of deterioration in mood. It was also suggested that patients who fail to seek support during such an episode may be less likely to keep up a positive mood in the face of increased pain.

It is hardly surprising that health professionals encounter a wide variation of emotional and behavioural responses to pain. Guidance and support to help a person feel in control can be very useful (see Chapters 8 and 9 for further discussion).

Other psychological factors

People who have a tendency towards hysterical or obsessional behaviour may respond to pain in a variety of ways which can bring them into conflict with medical or nursing staff. This may present problems, especially when staff expect patients to conform to an expected pattern of behaviour. Sometimes the term 'supra-tentorial' is used when referring to patients whose pain is not thought to have a physical basis. The use of this term may be a way of avoiding clear thinking and dismissing any pain the speaker does not feel is 'justified' – anything from conversion hysteria to an extreme reaction to pain because of fear. Health professionals should be aware of the use of this term and guard against being taken in by it. Another point of particular note when considering psychological factors is the influence of fatigue. With prolonged pain, the patient gets more tired and there is an accompanying lowering of pain threshold.

Psychological factors play such an important part in pain perception and expression that sometimes a patient may be labelled by carers as having pain which is 'psychogenic'. This term is controversial and it is most important that the term 'psychogenic pain' is reserved for patients who have absolutely no physical finding and a definite psychological history of expressing emotional problems in terms of pain (Sternbach, 1982). True psychogenic pain is a rare phenomenon. One reason it is encountered in the literature may be because medical techniques sometimes fail. It should be noted that for most patients experiencing chronic pain, the pain has an underlying physical basis, with emotional and behavioural factors contributing in varying degrees to the perception and expression of pain. It has been shown that it is more usual for a psychological disturbance to be the result of chronic pain than the cause of it and that psychological manifestations may disappear after successful treatment of the pain (Sternbach and Timmermans, 1975).

Another factor which may play an important part in how people react to pain is their prior experiences of it and how it was managed previously. Both patients who told their stories in Chapter 1 would not relish the possibility of further hospitalizations. Walmsley, Brockopp and Brockopp (1992) reported that past pain experiences had a very strong influence on expectation of pain.

Psychiatric illness

A number of psychiatric illnesses such as depression and schizophrenia have pain as a symptom. If the psychiatric illness is treated successfully, the pain will often disappear. It is necessary, though, for the patient to have a psychiatric evaluation and appropriate psychiatric treatment. Sometimes patients are referred to a pain clinic where this evaluation may not be available.

Implications of psychological factors for nursing

As far as nursing implications are concerned, it is important to try to identify how people are coping and what information would be helpful to individual patients as part of preparation for surgery or other potentially painful events, in order to help them to cope. It should be noted, however, that the mental and emotional state of a patient can vary with time and that this may have an effect on severity, tolerance and expression of pain.

Pain may be seen unconsciously by patients as punishment, as a symbol of rejection or as a way of asking for help. Just as it may be a warning to the body, so it may be interpreted as a warning to the personality. Most often, pain is perceived as a threat to body image, producing anxiety. The nurse must be aware of signs of anxiety which may manifest as restlessness, avoidance of discussion or hostility (sometimes labelled as unco-operativeness). The nurse should respond with understanding to such situations, as defensiveness may increase a patient's stress.

It is often difficult to identify sources of psychological stress in patients, particularly in those suffering chronic pain. Chronic pain potentially has an impact on every aspect of a sufferer's life. It is not just the pain which is the problem but the sequelae (Wall, 1983). Using a method of assessment devised by Walker (Walker *et al.*, 1990), Walker and Sofaer (1998) found, in a small study of patients attending pain clinics, that it was possible to identify a number of variables associated with psychological distress in patients who suffered chronic pain. There was a combination of factors including: fears about the future, regrets about the past, age (younger people were more distressed), practical help (the more help the more distress), feeling unoccupied and personal relationship difficulties. The method provides a simple and quick way of assessing sources of psychological distress in chronic pain patients and may be useful to health professionals (particularly nurses) in such situations.

THE EFFECT OF LEARNING ON PAIN

The role that psychology plays in the pain experience of an individual is a complex one, dependent on physical or psychiatric illness, early life experiences, present environment, the meaning attached to pain and cultural background. These factors add up to the learning experience which colours the patient's attitude towards his pain. The reader might like to try the following exercise to illustrate the effect of learning on pain.

Close your eyes for a few minutes and think back to your early childhood. Try to recall a situation where you experienced a painful event – perhaps you fell off your bike and hurt your knee or you may have burnt your fingers in a pot of hot water. Recall if you can the reaction of a person who was with you or near you at the time – was it panic, anger, love or ridicule? What action was taken? How did you feel afterwards? Try doing this recall with some of your colleagues and compare experiences and reactions. Early experiences such as these, as well as parental behaviour, colour a person's future attitude towards pain. Together, these experiences constitute a patient's 'pain autobiography'.

So it is with patients facing stressful events; each person has a different learning experience to bring to his own situation. Skevington (1995) notes that people hold different theories, 'schemata', which guide them in selecting and absorbing knowledge and from this they make sense of their experiences.

Modelling

One aspect of learning is known as modelling (Bandura, 1971). This refers to the idea that a person can anticipate the behavioural consequences of a situation through observing others, without having to experience it himself. Thus, he may subsequently base his reaction to his own experience on the behaviour of those he has observed. Patients may or may not express pain according to the social modelling that goes on in an environment they find themselves, such as a ward. However, patients do learn to lean on each other for support and for strategies of pain control. It is not uncommon for patients to say, 'Everybody is in the same boat'. Nevertheless, if a patient does not verbally express his pain and behaves as the 'social norms' of a hospital ward dictate, it does not necessarily mean that his pain is being relieved. This is exemplified in a comment overheard from a staff nurse:

> He was sitting at the end of the ward watching television with the other patients. He didn't look in pain. But when his visitors arrived his wife came and asked for painkillers for him. He was just seeking attention!

Could it not simply have been one of several other scenarios? He didn't feel pain when the nurse saw him; his wife recognized he was in pain and wanted to help him or he was reluctant to ask for help himself in front of other patients who were being brave.

CULTURAL FACTORS

General observations of similarity in behaviour between members of the same ethnic group in relation to pain have led to the idea that cultural factors are an important consideration in the management of pain. In some cultures, rituals which we may associate with extreme discomfort seem to cause no trouble for the people involved, whereas in others, apparently trivial stimuli produce a marked response. Research has shown that pain tolerance levels do indeed vary from one cultural background to another (Sternbach and Turskey, 1965). For example, people of Anglo-Saxon origin tend to accept pain in a matter-of-fact way, whereas people with a Mediterranean background were found to be more expressive of their pain (Zborowski, 1969).

Anglo-Saxon culture tends to favour a high tolerance for pain although, as in any cultural group, tolerance varies greatly from one patient to another and also in the same patient in different situations. For example, a patient may be willing to tolerate pain while his family is visiting so that he can communicate with them but he is not willing to endure the same degree of pain at other times or, as in the anecdote related above, visiting time may bring much-needed relief.

Some patients refuse pain relief because they have a high pain tolerance, whereas others are not willing to endure any pain for any period of time. Sometimes staff place a value judgement on a patient's tolerance without realizing that this is a patient's own unique response to pain and that he or she is entitled to such a response. If a patient is a member of an ethnic minority, this could lead to unwarranted judgement of future patients from the same minority group, which could obstruct effective pain management. Ethnic background has been seen to influence the degree of inferred suffering. Among six ethnic groups studied, Jewish patients were consistently rated by nurses as having the greatest physical pain and the greatest psychological distress (Davitz and Davitz, 1975). The researchers also concluded that it is important to recognize that belief systems about suffering exist, because these systems have a potential influence on interactions between patients and nurses insofar as nurses may have preconceived notions or expectations regarding the pain and psychological distress of patients. Davitz and Davitz also reported an instance where one nurse mentioned her reaction to an 'Oriental' patient who was crying in a casualty department. The nurse had observed stoicism in 'Oriental' patients previously, and felt taken aback when she was confronted with someone who did not fulfil her expectations.

It is difficult to draw conclusions from the literature on ethnicity and pain. This is because there are differences also within ethnic groups (for example in terms of personality, clinical conditions and acculturation). However, Faucett, Gordon and Levine (1994) noted that in studies reporting experimental pain, northern European or Caucasian groups of people were often reported to have higher pain tolerance than other racial or ethnic groups. In their own study of postoperative dental pain, Faucett, Gordon and Levine (1994) found that patients of European descent reported less severe pain than those of black American or Latino descent. Regardless of ethnic group, they found that men in their study reported less severe pain than women. This finding was in line with experimental (non-clinical) studies, but not with an earlier study reported by Weisenberg *et al.* in 1975, where no ethnic differences were found for pain severity in patients with dental emergencies. Faucett, Gordon and Levine suggested that in line with other researchers (Lipton and Marbach, 1984; Bates, Edwards and Anderson, 1993), it would be erroneous to stereotype patients in pain on the basis of their ethnicity because of intraethnic variations and other behaviour related to pain expression.

Although there are obvious problems in carrying out crosscultural research (linguistic representations of pain being a major one), Weisenberg (1982) stated that the nature of research into cultural aspects of pain does allow a number of theoretical processes to be described in the acquisition and transference of cultural reactions to pain. Greenwald (1991) found that despite a high degree of assimilation that had occurred among ethnic groups in the USA, cultural background still had an effect on the expression of pain. He suggested that ethnicity of patients should continue to concern those who care for people in pain. Davis (1998) explores some of the ways in which culture influences people's perceptions and behaviours in relation to health and illness.

The meaning of pain

There is evidence to suggest that people attach meaning to their pain, which may influence the intensity and duration of the pain they feel and their readiness to accept or refuse medication. Some people may consider that the pain they are suffering is a form of punishment they must endure for past misdeeds, while others may say, 'What have I done to deserve this?'. A patient may refuse drugs because he believes they are a crutch, thinking that succumbing to sickness is a sign of weakness and that self-respect can be maintained by rejecting help (Amarasingham, 1980). Patients who believe in certain systems or values may be resistant to accepting advice. For example, Puerto Ricans in New York classified food, medicines and bodily states according to whether they were hot or cold. Hot substances were used to treat cold conditions and vice versa. Rashes and diarrhoea were considered hot and should therefore be treated with cool foods or medicines (Harwood, 1971).

PSYCHOLOGICAL SUPPORT OF PATIENTS IN PAIN BY NURSES

Suggestions

- Develop a relationship with a patient which gives the patient an opportunity to discuss his feelings and the meaning attached to pain.
- Try to find out from the patient how he sees himself in terms of personality. This will give you some clues as to how he may be helped to cope with stress and/or pain.
- Provide the patient with information about what he will experience in terms of hospital routines and procedures.
- Discuss with the patient how he feels about analgesia. For example, does he have any coping strategies of his own which he would like to try out? Emphasize the availability of pain relief as part of nursing care.
- Involve the patient as a partner in this effort and not as a dependant. In this way you will give him a sense of control. For the patient, this sense of control, both in acute and chronic pain, may decrease pain intensity and improve the quality of the patient's life. Many psychological strategies taught to patients, such as relaxation, are aimed at providing greater control over pain. Relaxation is discussed in Chapter 8.

Allowing for individual variation

There is a great danger of stereotyping patients. Nurses and other health professionals must make allowances for individual variations in relation to pain expression and the response to various therapies. Above all, labelling patients as 'good' or 'bad', 'co-operative' or 'unco-operative' must be avoided.

There are millions of unique individuals in the world. We have to accept that there are innumerable combinations of personality, childhood experience and cultural background. Our response must be to individualize pain relief. This means accepting what the patient tells us. It also means that the patient may experience difficulty telling us. Pain is difficult to express.

Scarry (1985) wrote about the vulnerability of the human body and she noted the inexpressibility of pain: not only the difficulty of describing pain but its ability to destroy a person's language. 'Whatever pain achieves, it achieves in part through its unsharability, and it ensures this unsharability through its resistance to language.' It is because of this that much research has focused on the creation of diagnostic tools to help patients express pain. The most notable of these is the McGill Pain Questionnaire (see Melzack and Wall, 1996).

The individual nature of pain is described below in the exact words of a man who experienced phantom limb pain for 47 years.

There is no method to accurately describe pain. Various words used, such as itch, tender, ache, discomfort, sore, agonizing, searing, burning, shooting, excruciating, really convey little understanding to the listener. They may be understatements, exaggerations or the wrong use of terms. Most phenomena have a common universal method of measurement, such as sound, wind velocity, earthquake intensity, and so on. But no sufferer can tell a doctor how much pain he is suffering, nor can a doctor measure it. Assuming that a reliable method is made available, the next problem would be the effect of pain of the same intensity on different individuals. Some would be incapacitated with, say, a figure of four; others would be able to function.

References

Amarasingham, L. R. (1980) Social and cultural perspectives on medication refusal. *American Journal of Psychiatry*, **137**, 353–8.

Bandura, A. (1971) Analysis of modeling processes, in *Psychological Modeling*, (ed. A. Bandura), Aldine-Atherton, New York.

Bates, M. S., Edwards, W. T. and Anderson K. O. (1993) Ethnocultural influences on variation in chronic pain perception. *Pain*, **52**, 101–12.

Bond, M. R. (1979) *Pain: Its Nature Analysis and Treatment*, Churchill Livingstone, Edinburgh.

Bond, M. R. and Pearson, I. B. (1969) Psychological aspects of pain in women with advanced cancer of the cervix. *Journal of Psychosomatic Research*, **13**, 13–19.

Boore, J. (1977) Preoperative care of patients. *Nursing Times*, **73**, (12), 409–11.

Brown, G. K. and Nicassio, P. M. (1987). Development of a questionnaire for the assessment of active and passive coping strategies in chronic pain patients. *Pain*, **31**, 53–64.

Carr, E. (1997) Managing post-operative pain: problems and solutions, in *Pain. Its Nature and Management*, (ed. V. N. Thomas), Baillière Tindall, London.

Casten, R. J., Parmelee, P. A., Kleban, M. H., Lawton, M. P. and Katz I. R. (1995). The relationship among anxiety, depression, and pain in a geriatric institutionalized sample. *Pain*, **61**, 271–6.

Craig, K. D. and Best, J. A. (1977) Perceived control over pain: individual differences and situational determinants. *Pain*, **3**, 127–35.

Crisson, J. E. and Keefe, F. J. (1988) The relationship of locus of control to pain coping strategies and psychological distress in chronic pain patients. *Pain*, **46**, 161–71.

Davis, B. (1998) Cultural dimensions of pain, in *Perspectives on Pain: Mapping the Territory*, (ed. B. Carter), Edward Arnold, London, Sydney, Auckland.

Davis, P. S. (1988) Changing nursing practice for more effective control of postoperative pain through a staff initiated educational programme. *Nurse Education Today*, **8**, 325–31.

Davitz, L. J. and Davitz, J. R. (1975) How nurses view patient suffering. *RN*, **38**(10), 6972–4.

Faucett, J., Gordon, N. and Levine. J. (1994) Differences in postoperative pain severity among four ethnic groups. *Journal of Pain and Symptom Management*, **9**(6), 383–9.

Fernandez, E. and Turk, D. C. (1995) The scope and significance of anger in the experience of chronic pain. *Pain*, **61**, 165–75.

Folkman, S. and Lazarus, R. S.(1980) An analysis of coping in a middle-aged community sample. *Journal of Health and Social Behaviour*, **21**, 219–39.

Greenwald, H. P. (1991) Interethnic differences in pain perception. *Pain*, **44**, 157–63.

Harwood, A. (1971) The hot–cold theory of disease: implications for treatment of Puerto Rican patients. *Journal of the American Medical Association*, **216**, 1153–8.

Hayward, J. (1975) *Information, a Prescription Against Pain*, RCN, London.

Janis, I. L. (1958) *Psychological Stress*. Wiley, Chichester.

Jensen, M. P., Karoly, P. and Harris, P. (1991) Assessing the affective component of chronic pain: development of the pain discomfort scale. *Journal of Psychosomatic Research*, **35**, 149–54.

Jensen, M. P., Turner, J. A., Romano, J. M. and Karoly, P. (1991) Coping with chronic pain: a critical review of the literature. *Pain*, **47**(3), 248–83.

Johnson, J. E., Dabbs, J. M. and Leventhall, H. (1970) Psychological factors in the welfare of surgical patients. *Nursing Research*, **19**, 18–29.

Keefe, F. J., Affleck, G., Starr, K., Caldwell, D. S. and Tennen, H. (1997) Pain coping strategies and coping efficacy in rheumatoid arthritis: a daily process analysis. *Pain*, **69**, 35–42.

Lipton, J. A. and Marbach, J. J. (1984) Ethnicity and the pain experience. *Social Science and Medicine*, **19**, 1279–98.

Melzack, R. and Wall, P. D. (1996) *The Challenge of Pain*, Penguin Books, London.

Nichols, M. K., Wilson, P. H. and Goyen, J. (1992) Comparison of cognitive-behavioural group treatment and an alternative non-psychological treatment for chronic low back pain. *Pain*, **48**, 339–47.

Romano, J. M. and Turner, J. A. (1985) Chronic pain and depression: does the evidence support the relationship? *Psychological Bulletin*, **97**, 18–34.

Rosenstiel, A. K. and Keefe, F. J. (1983) The use of coping strategies in chronic back pain patients: relationship to patient characteristics and current adjustment. *Pain*, **17**, 33–44.

Scarry, E. (1985) *The Body in Pain*, Oxford University Press, Oxford.

Skevington, S. M. (1995) *Psychology of Pain*, Wiley, Chichester.

Snow-Turek, A. L., Norris, M. P. and Tan, G. (1996) Active and passive coping strategies in chronic pain patients. *Pain*, **64**, 455–62.

Sternbach, R. A. (1982) The psychologist's role in the diagnosis and treatment of pain patients, in *Psychological Approaches to the Management of Pain*, (eds J. Barber and C. Adrian), Brunner Mazel, New York.

Sternbach, R. A. and Timmermans, G. (1975) Personality changes associated with reduction of pain. *Pain*, **1**, 177–81.

Sternbach, R. A. and Turskey, B. (1965) Ethnic differences in psychophysical and skin potential responses to electric shock. *Psychophysiology*, **1**, 241-6.

Taylor, A. G., Skelton, J. and Butcher, J. (1983) Duration of pain, condition and physical pathology: determinants of nurses' assessments of patients in pain. *Nursing Research*, **33**, 4–8.

Vingoe, F. J. (1994) Anxiety and pain: terrible twins or supportive siblings? in *Psychology, Pain and Anaesthesia*, (ed. H. B. Gibson), Stanley Thornes (Publishers) Ltd, Cheltenham.

Wade, J., Price, D. D., Hamer, R. M., Schwartz, S. M. and Hart, R. P. (1990) An emotional component analysis of chronic pain. *Pain*, **40**(3), 303–10.

Walker, J. M. and Sofaer, B. (1998) Predictors of psychological stress in chronic pain patients. *Journal of Advanced Nursing*, **27**, 320–6.

Walker, J. M., Akinsanya, J. A., Davis, B. D. and Marcer, D. (1990) The nursing management of patients in the community: a theoretical framework. *Journal of Advanced Nursing*, **14**, 240–7.

Wall, P. D. (1983) Pain as a 'need state'. *Journal of Psychosomatic Research*, **27**, 413.

Walmsley, P. N. H., Brockopp, D. Y. and Brockopp, G. W. (1992) The role of prior pain experience and expectations on post-operative pain. *Journal of Pain and Symptom Management*, **7**, 34–7.

Weisenberg. M. (1982) Cultural and ethnic factors in reaction to pain, in *Culture and Psychopathology*, (ed. I. Al Issa), University Park Press, Baltimore.

Weisenberg, M., Kreindler, M. L., Schachat, R. and Werboff, J. (1975) Pain: anxiety and attitudes in black, white and Puerto Rican patients. *Psychosomatic Medicine*, **37**, 123–35.

Zborowski, M. (1969) *People in Pain*. Jossey-Bass, San Diego.

Beliefs, responsibility, educational issues and communication

4

I envy for our medical students the advantages enjoyed by the nurses who live in daily contact with the sick.

Osler, 1947

In this chapter some beliefs of health professionals are explored. The issue of responsibility and partnership is addressed, the need for education is emphasized and finally the problem of communication between patients and health professionals and between health professionals themselves is discussed.

BELIEFS AND VALUES

Nurses, more than other health professionals, have the opportunity to develop close and fulfilling professional relationships with patients. In this respect, nurses are in a unique position to assess the physical and psychological well-being of patients, especially in response to treatment, and to communicate this information to each other, their medical colleagues and other members of the caring team. This is in no way meant to imply that other members of the health care team do not also have responsibilities. Doctors, physiotherapists and other people who care for patients should be able to relate to patients in a way that indicates that they are aware of pain and the importance of managing it effectively.

As discussed in Chapter 3, a patient brings to each painful situation his past experiences of pain, experiences coloured not only by his own personality but by the behaviour of those around him at the time. However, the patient is not alone in bringing a pain autobiography to a current situation, since those who care for him also have pain autobiographies. In some situations this might be of help to a patient but in others it may not. For example, a nurse who has suffered pain herself is likely to have a greater understanding of a patient's pain than one who has not, while a nurse brought up to believe in a 'grin-and-bear-it' attitude towards pain might not find it easy to empathize with a patient. We may know what is happening to a patient in the physiological sense but seldom do we know what it feels like.

A patient who comes into hospital is thus faced with a team of carers who may have different attitudes and values in relation to pain, its expression and control. In British hospital wards, the nurse is the key person whose attitudes and beliefs influence whether or not a patient receives the best possible pain relief, first through her reports to the medical staff about the patient and, second, because of her responsibility for interpreting administration times for drugs or other thera- pies. The danger is one of interpreting a patient's needs in accordance with set rou- tines of a particular health-care setting or ward or holding inbuilt personal values about pain. Of course, patients' needs are as individual as they themselves are and pain relief should be administered accordingly. Unfortunately, however, research findings have shown that nurses and patients may not agree about the severity of patients' pain (Seers, 1989). Sofaer (1984) found that only 9% of nurses (n = 64) felt that the aim of administering analgesics during the first two postoperative days was to relieve pain completely, compared with 28% of patients (n = 87).

PERSONAL JUDGEMENTS

Nurses may make personal judgements of patients' suffering based on their own beliefs. The following extract is quoted from Davitz and Davitz (1975) and illus- trates how feelings and behaviour were affected as a result of personal judge- ments.

On the unit, she [the nurse] attended two mothers. One had a normal healthy baby girl and the other gave birth to a boy with a cleft palate. Both mothers reacted negatively to the births. The mother of the baby girl had wanted a boy. She was hysterical, refused to see the infant and became withdrawn and hostile. The mother of the baby with a cleft palate displayed equally violent reactions. She, too, rejected all contact with the infant and staff. The nurse reacted to the mother of the baby who had a cleft palate with great sympathy and understand- ing. 'I went in to see her and no matter what she said or did, I knew I had to stay and help. She needed us, though she fought against all the help we tried to give.' The mother of the girl received routine care. 'It drove us up a wall to hear this woman carrying on the way she did. She was lucky she had a healthy baby. For her to complain didn't make sense. All of us could understand the feelings of the woman who had a baby with a cleft palate – but this woman kind of made us angry. None of us felt like rushing in to see her when she called.'

Each of the patients felt distressed. From the mothers' points of view, the psychological strain of the disappointing births might have been comparable. However, from the nurse's point of view the situations differed. The two women simply weren't seen as suffering the same degree of psychological distress. The nurse's reactions were not determined by differences in the behaviour of the two women. As a matter of fact, the two mothers apparently behaved in very much the same way. Thus, it was not the patients' behaviour that made the difference, but the nurse's beliefs about suffering. She didn't believe that the mother who was disappointed with the sex of her baby could suffer as much as the mother of a baby born with a cleft palate. The crucial difference in the matter, therefore, was the nurse's system of beliefs about suffering.

In *RN, The Full-Service Nursing Journal*, 1975. QC Medical Economics Company Inc., Oracle, NJ. Reprinted with permission.

The same authors studied nurses' inferences of suffering by asking nurses to rate the degree of physical pain and degree of psychological distress of patients suffering from 15 different illnesses and injuries. They found that nurses have some common beliefs about suffering.

Results show that a patient's socio-economic status, age, and ethnic background are important determinants of the amount of suffering likely to be inferred by a nurse. For example, lower-class patients were generally seen as suffering greater physical pain than middle or upper-class patients. For instance, an unskilled labourer with thrombophlebitis was seen as experiencing greater pain than either a teacher or bank president of the same age and sex. Nurses saw male and female patients suffering equivalent degrees of physical pain and psychological distress. However, when sex was considered in relationship to social class, the fact that a patient was male or female did make a difference. For example, lower-class women were seen as suffering more physical pain than lower-class men who had the same illnesses or injuries and were the same age. However, the reverse was true for upper-class women and men. Upper-class women were seen as suffering less physical pain than upper-class men.

Bringing prior knowledge (rather than prejudice) to a situation may be helpful. For example, if a certain illness is usually very painful, then one can be on the lookout for signs of distress. Nevertheless, as already pointed out, we should be aware of the dangers of stereotyping because it can lead to misunderstandings. It is important that health professionals examine their own beliefs and values about suffering and learn to be on their guard for misperceptions and misunderstandings.

There are reports in the literature that patients who complain of pain or discomfort are seen as 'bad' patients (Lorber, 1975; Raps *et al.*, 1982). Johnson (1982) found that 'being liked' by nurses was important to patients and Salmon and Manyande (1996) found that nurses overestimated patients' ability to cope with pain and those who displayed bad coping or displayed distress were unpopular with nurses. Thorn (1997) found that nurses held misplaced beliefs in relation to the relief of postoperative pain. These included such issues as the patient's right to be pain free and nurses believing that they had to 'verify' the patient's report of pain.

INCONGRUENCE OF BELIEFS AND VALUES WITHIN THE TEAM OF HEALTH PROFESSIONALS

It is not uncommon for members of a team of health professionals to disagree on how best to provide pain relief for a particular patient. It is sometimes found that the more junior staff are more compassionate towards patients, but unfortunately also the most powerless. Students of nursing frequently report that they want to help patients but feel 'powerless'.

The patient who is in pain just wants relief. Nurses who are not in a position to sanction relief, or request review of analgesic requirements by the doctor because of their lack of seniority, can be made to feel helpless. (Chapter 5 stresses the importance of assessment which can help to relieve the helplessness of a nurse.) It is not uncommon for junior nurses to apologize to patients by saying something like, 'I'm afraid you're not due your painkillers yet' or 'The drug trolley will be around in half an hour'. If a patient reports pain to a nurse before the time when medication is due according to the prescription, then the nurse in charge *must* consider it her responsibility to inform the doctor with a view to increasing the efficacy of the medication. Doctors rely on nursing colleagues to report patients' pain because they themselves cannot be on hand 24 hours a day to assess patients' individual requirements. Likewise, if a patient reports a side effect of a drug or a symptom which could be a side effect then the nurse must contact a doctor for advice. The following example is illustrative of such a situation:

A young student was hospitalized with acute follicular tonsillitis. She hadn't eaten much for the past two or three days prior to being admitted to hospital and was receiving intravenous antibiotics. She was given a 'pink medicine' for the pain in her throat. The medicine was effective but she complained of nausea and abdominal pain shortly after each administration of the 'pink medicine'. Nobody paid attention. Her mother (a trained nurse) was concerned and enquired casually as to what the medicine was. On learning that it was Voltarol, the mother said: 'My daughter is reporting gastric irritation', to which the staff nurse replied (with the most extraordinary non-verbal communication of shutting her eyes), 'Most unusual in someone her age'. Clearly, the nurse was unaware that gastric irritation is to do with gastric mucosal response and is not age related!

RESPONSES TO AND EXPECTATIONS OF PATIENTS' BEHAVIOUR

Sometimes nurses' concern about a patient's distress is related to the medical diagnosis or to the type of operation the patient has had. For example, pain following minor surgery may be dismissed because of the simplicity of the surgical technique involved, whereas someone who has undergone a more complicated surgical procedure may attract more attention. The nurse, without paying attention to what the patient is experiencing, may feel that the latter type of operation should result in more pain. One ex-patient, herself a nurse, reported pain in her chest to the nursing staff on her admission to hospital. No pain relief or sympathy was forthcoming until a diagnosis had been made.

Illnesses or procedures have different meanings for different people and these may affect their pain behaviour. For example, someone may be so relieved at undergoing a hysterectomy following years of unpleasant symptoms that the postoperative pain may be much better tolerated than that experienced by a patient who has undergone another form of surgery but who has had no previous symptoms. One patient who had a hysterectomy declined much in the way of analgesics offered to her and disclosed that she had been 'beaten up' by her husband so frequently that the postoperative pain seemed meaningless in comparison. One should not have rigid expectations of the way a patient with a given condition should feel. For example, it is not helpful to make remarks such as, 'Mrs Jones had the same operation two days ago and she is up and about' or, prior to a procedure, 'You should be up and about in 24 hours'. If patients have difficulty in meeting these expectations they may feel a sense of failure.

Prejudice on the part of the health professional may be related to patient adaptation. In this situation a patient's pain may be less socially visible and the patient is consequently regarded with suspicion. Hackett (1971), a psychiatrist interested in treating patients in pain, noted:

> The individual stands before you in the examining room calmly and coolly describing the agony he is in and your first response is to doubt that he suffers as much as he claims.

Although this quotation is over 25 years old it still has relevance today. People describe pain in different ways and with varying degrees of visibility. One man in his 30s who suffered terrible injuries during an accident in an office, took aspirin for four days before going to a hospital to seek help. He was admitted at once when it was diagnosed that he had serious spinal injuries.

It is important to remember that whereas the patient may have adapted his behaviour, the pain may remain at the same intensity. In relation to painful procedures, sometimes doctors and nurses say, 'You won't feel anything' or 'This will hurt a little' or 'It shouldn't be that sore'. It would be more helpful to patients if something along the following lines was said: 'This may be painful for some people – let me know how it is for you'. In this way, the patient is not embarrassed into conforming with expectations of him and is allowed to express his own experience.

Both the efficacy and duration of action of a drug can vary from one patient to another. This problem is often compounded by standard prescription frameworks such as the 'magic' four-hourly regime. Nurses often expect patients' behaviour to conform to this regime. Sometimes, if patients manage to conform, they are labelled 'awfully good' while if they do not, they are labelled as 'unco-operative' or 'complaining'. One staff nurse said, 'Before I learnt about the individual nature of pain, I classified patients according to their operations and expected them to behave alike in relation to their pain relief requirements'.

LEARNING ABOUT PAIN RELIEF

Perhaps the most significant factor contributing to lack of awareness of the importance of pain relief among health carers is the lack of education on the subject of pain and its relief in student curricula. Since man's fear of pain is associated with his fear of death (Sternbach, 1968), this lamentable situation must be remedied both during basic training and by post-basic continuing education programmes. Lack of education could be a primary problem faced by nursing staff when trying to help patients in pain. Sofaer (1984) found that only 14% of nurses felt themselves to be well prepared, 75% would have liked more education, and 11% felt themselves to be badly prepared. Twelve years on, Clarke *et al.* (1996) highlighted knowledge deficits and inconsistent responses in many areas related to pain management with patients.

Trained nurses act as models for less experienced nurses. If trained staff are poorly informed on current research and theory in relation to pain and its relief, then the status quo of lack of knowledge and ill-founded myths will continue. One staff nurse commented, 'For years I've been handing out analgesics, never thinking about whether they were effective or not or how long they lasted'.

If a nurse is well informed on aspects of pain management, she could use the combination of her unique position as a carer, together with her knowledge, to increase her own confidence and to communicate better with medical colleagues to ensure that patients don't suffer. There again, if medical students were taught more about the importance of pain relief they would presumably take the issue on board.

The International Association for the Study of Pain's publication of the Core Curriculum for Professional Education in Pain (1991) was an important step forward. As far as nurses are concerned, many feel the need for education but despite this, basic nursing education appears to devote little time to pain (Franke, Garssen and Abu-Saad, 1996) and there is mounting evidence that pain is not well relieved. (Graffam, 1990; Davis, 1991; Diekmann and Wassem, 1991). According to Sofaer (1984) education is more effective when it is ward based and is directed to all members of the nursing team. Franke, Garssen and Abu-Saad (1996) examined 12 studies of educational programmes on pain management for nurses and concluded that they can have an impact on both nurses and patients.

ACCOUNTABILITY VERSUS POWER

Pain relief tends to be a low priority. For whatever reason – the lack of education or perhaps the organization of the system – members of health-care teams do not always hold themselves or each other accountable for relieving pain. Doctors write prescriptions and nurses administer analgesics, but nurses may not question in their own minds the efficacy or suitability of a medication for a particular patient and may be reluctant to report any shortcomings of the treatment to the doctor. If nurses do not involve themselves, the doctors' task will be made extremely difficult and sometimes impossible.

It sometimes seems that we are more concerned about minimizing patients' expression of pain than the pain itself. (After McCaffery, 1983.)

A patient recalled how he had lost control. He was in pain but felt he had to put on a brave face at first.

I asked nicely for some pain relief but the staff were busy and the pain got worse. I felt I wanted to bang my fist against something. I shouted at the nurse, 'Get me something for this bloody pain'. Later that evening the sister came to me and said 'I hear you were rude to the staff nurse, she is very upset'. I felt I had to apologize. But I felt resentful. I had been in such pain and they had left me.

Another patient's comments again illustrate how sometimes analgesia is prescribed but not forthcoming when patients need it.

Once or twice I asked a nurse for tablets for the pain or for something to help me when I felt sick, but an hour or so later I was still waiting. Nobody ever came near me and I didn't know whether to ask them for anything again because nobody seemed to bother. You could ask a nurse something and she'd say, 'Right, I'll go and get sister' but nothing happened and you still weren't any better off. So half the time I thought there wasn't any point in asking them.

Staff often appear to control patients' expression of pain. A patient may be encouraged to 'get hold of himself' or 'not disturb other patients'. Sometimes a patient may feel uncomfortable about 'bothering the nurse' because he has been told he can only have medication at certain times. This can be a particular problem at night when pain may keep him awake. It is not unknown for nurses to report that a patient had a 'good night' but for the patient to report that pain kept him awake.

On the other hand, it can be very rewarding to see pain being relieved when analgesia is quickly forthcoming, as in the following example. A young woman returned from the operating theatre and on coming round from the anaesthetic, reported 'agony'. The staff were surprised, as normally analgesia was given routinely in the recovery room. Within two minutes of the patient reporting pain, they administered morphine and the patient had good relief.

PARTNERSHIP

Patients may sometimes be suffering in silence. This seems to be the case particularly when people are in acute pain. The issue of accountability for pain relief is therefore most important for the nursing profession. Being accountable means realizing that we must share in a partnership with each patient. If a partnership exists, then the patient has a right to judge if the care is satisfactory. The pain is the patient's subjective experience.

Partnership is not 'powership'. Partnership means that there is equality, an openness to suggestions and acceptance of responsibility by the parties involved. In the management of chronic pain, there needs to be involvement of the family if the person experiencing the pain is expected to relinquish bad habits. The family will also have become adjusted to the life of pain.

Nurses and other health professionals should be able to offer the patient the opportunity to choose what treatment may suit him best. This requires having a wide knowledge of treatments and coping strategies. More particularly, it requires attitudes that allow patients to have control over their own pain and to maintain their self-respect. Patients should be encouraged not to feel that they must inevitably suffer pain. The way in which nursing care is organized may influence how nurses can exercise accountability. The way medical care is organized so often means confidence or lack of it on the part of the patient. Not everybody can achieve an excellent relationship. When a nurse or a doctor finds a situation such as this they should consult a colleague so that attempts can be made to help the patient. Nobody gets it right all the time.

Nurses have a special part to play

It is important to be aware that trust, respect and empathy are essential to good communication. One reason why pain control may not be achieved is failure on the part of the nurse to realize that she has an important part to play. On the other hand, a nurse may realize the importance of her own role, but the process of communication with others may present difficulties. This might occur because of the organizational setting or, as mentioned earlier, because a nurse brings her own subjective experiences to the situation. In hospital settings, staff take for granted the day-to-day routines and this may blind them to some of the important aspects of interpersonal communication (Fagerhaugh and Strauss, 1977).

Within certain limits, a nurse can choose how she moulds the situation in which she finds herself. She can either make active efforts to change situations and circumstances for the benefit of patients or remain ambivalent. For example, in relation to the administration of analgesia, the nurse's interpretation of a prescription written four-hourly 'when necessary' can affect whether a patient suffers unnecessary pain or not. If the nurse interprets such a prescription to mean that she gives medication at the traditional drug round times only, she will deprive those patients whose requirements do not match her drug rounds. If, on the other hand, she assesses pain relief on an individual basis, patients are likely to benefit from pain control rather than pain relief; the implication here being that patients will be free from peaks of pain that occur as the effects of the drug wear off. Obviously, it takes time for each drug administration to have an effect, so patients could experience a considerable duration of pain if analgesia is only administered when pain becomes severe.

A further point is that nurses record when an analgesic drug or other pain relief measure has been administered but they seldom record the effect. Clarke *et al.*

(1996) found that even in a clinical setting where there were policies and resources in place regarding the management of pain they were not utilized enough. Nurses should record and report pain in much more detail than is often done. If this were the case, then at the end of each shift the information collected would be helpful to the new shift in ensuring good continuity of care. It is also important to note how long it takes for a dose of medication to have an effect, how much relief it provides with or without other pain-relieving strategies and how long the relief lasts. In addition, it is valuable to know how the medication was tolerated by the patient and essential to know of any adverse effects. This information is not only of help to nurses but of inestimable value to the medical staff.

Responsibility lies in the provision of humane caring in general and the concerned provision of adequate pain control in particular. This should be based on a relationship between patient and the carers which gives the patient 'space' to share in the decision making. To achieve this requires skilled communication between nursing colleagues, doctors and patients.

COMMUNICATION

Some patients do not express their pain verbally. We may not assume that pain is absent just because behaviour does not indicate its presence. People may be inhibited because of all sorts of reasons. This includes 'embarrassment' in acute pain and 'adaptation' in chronic pain.

Figure 4.1 is a simple diagrammatic representation of communication between nurse, doctor and a patient in pain. A depicts potential communication, and is shown by broken lines. B shows the patient not verbalizing her need for relief, the nurse 'not seeing' and the doctor 'not hearing'. In C, the patient is shown as pain free and smiling and the line of communication between the three people is unbroken.

Nurses and doctors

The interaction between nurses and doctors is of great importance in pain control. Sometimes relationships are less harmonious than they might be and expectations of each other may be unrealistic. Doctors rely on nurses for reports and nurses may be able to help the doctor to see the patient's point of view. Sometimes, however, nurses do not like to 'question' a doctor's judgement of a situation, yet no doctor would wish a patient to suffer and most welcome recognition by a nurse that analgesia is ineffective. The following anecdote (Sofaer, 1983b) illustrates a sad lack of communication.

A senior charge nurse complained that one of the anaesthetists had been prescribing the same amount of postoperative analgesia on a four-hourly 'as necessary' basis for 30 years. 'It's not a satisfactory arrangement', she said, 'Sometimes a patient requires the medication more frequently and at other times in an increased dose.' When asked why she could not simply request the doctor to be a little more flexible in his prescribing or request a change of prescription by the houseman, she said, 'It's hospital policy that the anaesthetist writes up the postoperative medication for the first 24 hours' and 'We've been working together for 30 years and it's impossible to fight with him'.

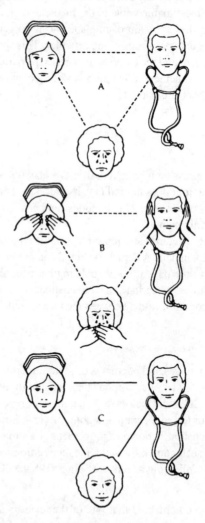

Figure 4.1 Diagrammatic representation of communication between nurse, doctor and a patient in pain. (A) potential communication; (B) non-communication; (C) successful communication. (Adapted with permission from Sofaer, 1987.)

It was suggested that she might try using a postoperative pain assessment chart and seeking the anaesthetist's assistance when analgesia was not effective. When the anaesthetist was told that the ward would be trying out an assessment chart, he said:

> That's a good idea. I always prescribe four-hourly 'as necessary' for the first 24 hours and I am always concerned that patients may suffer unnecessarily because the staff don't know how to interpret the prescription on the basis of individual needs. Nobody ever phones me! I've been working with the charge nurse for 30 years now and it would be quite impossible to tell her what to do.

Even after 30 years of poor communication between two professional people, both of whom 'cared' in their own way, it was possible to improve postoperative pain management by making the recording of pain more systematic. In addition, a teaching programme was implemented on the ward, aimed at increasing the knowledge and awareness of staff. This combined approach may have helped them towards increasing responsibility and accountability (Sofaer, 1983a).

The story may seem 'old hat' to a nurse working on wards where there is a system of pain assessment and where for surgical pain, patient-controlled analgesia is used. This may be the case but, even so, nurses still sometimes blame doctors and doctors sometimes blame nurses. It would be more helpful to find ways of communicating in an understanding way, recognizing that trust and respect are beneficial all round, especially to the patient.

Twycross and Lack (1983) have also emphasized the importance of teamwork in the relief of pain, particularly in terminal care, and although this is not addressed specifically in this book, the principles are no different when it comes to communication.

Patient information

One aspect of communication often important for patients' peace of mind is the need for doctors and nurses to explain, in terms that a patient understands, the physiological or pathological basis for pain. Patients may sometimes have mistaken ideas of the pathological processes involved and these can be more terrifying than the actual disease. For example two patients were very concerned about their future bladder function having undergone cholecystectomy. They thought that the gall bladder was part of the urinary system. Simple anatomical drawings or illustrations can obviously help to dispel such misconceptions. A brief summary of any explanation given can be written in the case notes and nursing care plan so that colleagues will be aware of what has been done and of any metaphor or analogy used.

In an outpatient setting it may be useful for the patient to have a tape recording made of the consultation to listen to when at home, alone, with family or friends. Sofaer and Lamberty (1995) reported how useful this was to patients in helping them to understand more about their chronic pain and possible treatments for it.

References

Clarke, E. B., French, B., Bilodeau, M. L. *et al.* (1996) Pain management knowledge, attitudes and clinical practice: the impact of nurses' characteristics and education. *Journal of Pain and Symptom Management*, **11**(1), 18–31.

Davis, P. S. (1991) Teaching nurses about managing pain. *Nursing Standard*, **5**(52), 30–3.

Davitz, L. J. and Davitz, J. R. (1975) How nurses view patient suffering. *RN*, **38**(10), 6972–4.

Diekmann, J. M. and Wassem, R. A. (1991) A survey of nursing students' knowledge of cancer pain control. *Cancer Nursing*, **14**(6), 314–19

Fagerhaugh, S. Y. and Strauss, A. (1977) *Politics of Pain Management: Staff–patient Interaction*, Addison-Wesley, New York.

Franke, A. L. Garssen, B. and Abu-Saad, H. H. (1996) Continuing pain education in nursing: a literature review. *International Journal of Nursing Studies*, **33**(5), 567–78.

Graffam, S. (1990) Pain content in the curriculum: a survey. *Nurse Education*, **15**, 20–3.

Hackett, T. P. (1971) Pain and prejudice: why do we doubt that the patient is in pain? *Medical Times*, **99**(2), 130–41.

International Association for the Study of Pain (1991) *Core Curriculum for Professional Education in Pain*, (ed. H. Field), IASP, Seattle.

Johnson, M. (1982) Recognition of patients' worries by nurses and by other patients. *British Journal of Clinical Psychology*, **21**, 255–61.

Lorber, J. (1975) Good patients and problem patients: conformity and deviance in a general hospital. *Journal of Health and Social Behaviour*, **16**, 213–25.

McCaffery, M. (1983) *Nursing the Patient in Pain*, Harper and Row, London.

Osler, W. (1947) *The Hospital as a College*, Blackstone, Aequanimatas.

Raps, C. S., Peterson, C., Jones, M. and Seligman, M. E. P. (1982) Patient behaviour in hospitals: helplessness, reactance or both? *Journal of Personal and Social Psychology*, **42**, 1036–41.

Salmon, P. and Manyande, A. (1996) Good patients cope with their pain: postoperative analgesia and nurses' perceptions of their patients' pain. *Pain*, **68**, 63–8.

Seers, K. (1989) Patients' perception of acute pain, in *Directions in Nursing Research*, (eds J. Wilson-Barnett and S. Robinson), Scutari Press, London, pp. 107–16.

Sofaer, B. (1983a) The effect of focused nursing education on postoperative pain relief: a pilot study, in *Proceedings of the First Open Conference of the Workgroup for European Nurse Researchers*, Swedish Nurses Association.

Sofaer, B. (1983b) Pain relief: the importance of communication. *Nursing Times*, **79**(48), 325.

Sofaer, B. (1984) The effect of focused education for nursing teams on postoperative pain of patients. Unpublished PhD thesis, University of Edinburgh.

Sofaer, B. (1987) Pain. Helping to meet the challenge from a nursing point of view, in *Nursing the Physically Ill Adult*, (eds J. R. P. Boore, R. Champion and M. C. Ferguson), Churchill Livingstone, Edinburgh.

Sofaer, B. (1992) *Pain: A Handbook for Nurses*, 2nd edn, Chapman and Hall, London.

Sofaer, B. and Lamberty, J. (1995) The use of taped consultations in the pain clinic. Poster for Pain in Europe,1st Scientific Meeting of the European Federation of IASP Chapters, Verona.

Sternbach, R. A. (1968) *Pain. A Psychophysiological Analysis*, Academic Press, New York.

Thorn, M. (1997) A survey of nurses' attitudes towards the assessment and control of post-operative pain. *Journal of Orthopaedic Nursing*, **1**(1), 1–54.

Twycross, R. G. and Lack, S. A. (1983) *Symptom Control in Far Advanced Cancer: Pain Relief*, Pitman Books, London.

5

Assessing pain

> When we can assess the patient's pain accurately, we can treat it more effectively.
>
> *McCaffery, 1983*

In this chapter on assessing pain, discussion is focused on the efforts of health professionals, particularly nurses, to assess pain with patients. The importance of recognizing individual coping strategies of patients, the constraints placed on patients' requests for pain relief and the value of having a written record which facilitates communication between patients, nurses and doctors will be emphasized.

The chapter does not relate assessment of pain to current 'models of nursing'. This is deliberate and is because pain is a subjective phenomenon and should not be related to or bound within prescriptive ideas which may not encompass all the factors which are necessary in good qualitative assessment. Human experience is wide ranging and any assessment of pain should be based on a humanistic perception of what is going on with a patient at the time he or she is suffering. Hardy (1990), in an excellent article arguing against the use of theoretical models, noted that human situations are complex and encouraged nurses to 'explore the mysteries' of their own work to improve the quality of the patient experience. The experience of pain is one which changes within each individual over time as well as being different in each individual. These experiences require what Hardy calls 'creative responses to new situations'.

This does not preclude the use of a tool to assist in assessment. Keeping a record can be helpful to both patients and staff. Ferrell (1991) made the point, that, although we are able to manage pain effectively using available innovations and tools, they are useless unless clinically applied. Dufault *et al.* (1995) identified barriers to using innovations in pain relief and they noted that one of these is lack of interest and understanding of research findings by practising nurses. But, as

Tanabe (1995) has pointed out, it is only through promotion of pain assessment that pain management will become a priority.

It is very clear from the literature and from anecdotal evidence that poor (or no) pain assessment practices exist widely (Camp and O'Sullivan, 1987; Seers, 1989; Harrison, 1991; Allcock, 1996).

Various explanations have been put forward for the lack of good pain assessment. Lander (1990) suggested that nurses who see a great deal of pain may become less impressed by it. Choiniere *et al.* (1990) speculated that because nurses were unable to manage pain effectively, they played down the levels of pain which patients experienced. Mackintosh (1994) found that 87% of nurses she interviewed in a study on postoperative pain felt that they underestimated levels of pain in patients.

'PAIN CUES'

The process of pain assessment requires active effort on the part of the nurse and must begin with the recognition that pain is a subjective experience. In order to provide relief for a patient, the nurse must be able to recognize 'pain cues' and to evaluate the extent of the suffering. The task is not an easy one and even very experienced nurses may underestimate the severity of a patient's pain.

One reason for the difficulty is that patients and nurses have varying values and beliefs about how one is expected to react to and report pain. For example, a nurse may expect a patient to show objective signs of pain. These may include elevated blood pressure, increased pulse and respiration rates and perspiration. She may expect a patient to communicate his pain verbally or to show signs of pain through non-verbal behaviour such as writhing or restlessness. However, although these cues may be present in some patients, lack of expressions of pain or lack of objective signs of pain does not necessarily mean lack of pain. Patients may adapt to pain both behaviourally and physiologically, perhaps because they place a high value on self-control, so that signs of suffering may be suppressed. Furthermore, because illness and pain are fatiguing, sometimes patients react by being quieter than usual and by lying still simply because they are too tired to do otherwise. It also could be that nurses expect others to control their feelings because they themselves have to do so in situations of stress (McCaffery, 1983).

One difficulty often voiced by nurses is in assessing the efficacy of analgesic drugs. If a patient reports pain prior to the time when the next dose of medication is due, he should not be made to feel that he is reacting in an inappropriate way. There is much evidence, particularly in relation to relief of postoperative pain, to suggest that undertreatment of patients is alarmingly common (Marks and Sachar, 1973; Cohen, 1980; Weis *et al.*, 1983). A patient's behaviour should not be thoughtlessly compared to that of other patients who have undergone the same or similar operations.

DIFFERENT RESPONSES TO PAIN

Some patients may show minimal response to pain because they have devised their own coping strategies for distracting themselves. Under certain circumstances, nurses may not fully appreciate that a patient is watching television, knitting or listening to music to take his mind off his pain. Often patients do not tell the staff about the methods they have devised to cope with pain, with the result that a decrease in pain expression may be misinterpreted by staff as meaning that pain has diminished or disappeared. For some patients, the expression of pain would make them feel ashamed or embarrassed.

Elderly people

Walker *et al.* (1990) have shown that for elderly patients suffering pain in the community, personal strategies were important in maintaining control over chronic pain. Thus, the assessment of patients' coping status could pave the way for more patient-centred care. Walker *et al.*'s assessment scheme for elderly patients is based on the wide literature on pain and care of the elderly patient, but could be utilized or adapted to meet the needs of many patients who suffer chronic pain (Figure 5.1). Weiner *et al.* (1996) suggested that 'pain behaviour observation' is a valid assessment tool in the elderly. Reviewing the literature on pain in elderly people, Gagliese and Melzack (1997) suggested that the majority of elderly people suffered pain of such intensity that it interfered with their normal functioning. They noted that because of concerns regarding possible adverse pharmacological treatments, pain relief in this group may be inadequate but that, like younger people, elderly people would benefit from non-pharmacological interventions. They noted that pain at a level which interferes with life is not a normal part of ageing. For further reading on pain in the elderly, see Walker (1993).

Pain tolerance

Pain tolerance is the intensity of pain that an individual is willing to accept without seeking relief. Sometimes patients are referred to by staff as having a low pain tolerance. This may be disapproved of by some nursing staff who themselves value stoicism and admire people with willpower. This judgement may interfere with a nurse's assessment of pain and militate against effecting relief. A person's ability to tolerate pain may be affected by the psychological and cultural factors discussed in Chapter 3, including anxiety level and past experiences. One example is the behaviour of a young international cello player who broke his wrist. Although the pain may have been considerable, his anxiety about being able to regain his finger movements again was foremost in his mind. He never once reported pain and during physiotherapy his main goal was regaining movement *no matter what*. His future career was so much at stake. His feelings were understood sympathetically by his doctors, nurses and music teachers.

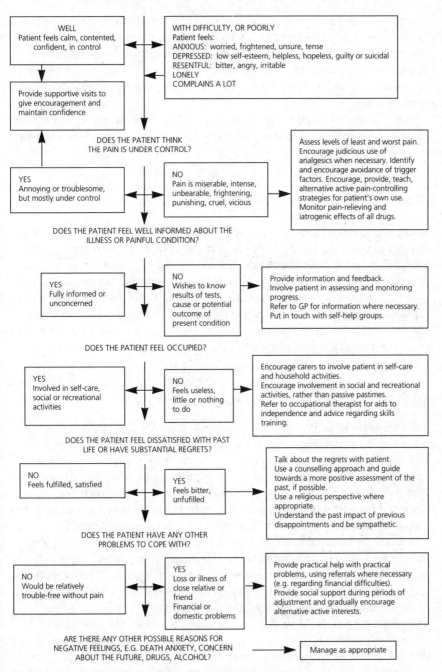

HOW IS THE PATIENT COPING?

WELL
Patient feels calm, contented, confident, in control

WITH DIFFICULTY, OR POORLY
Patient feels:
ANXIOUS: worried, frightened, unsure, tense
DEPRESSED: low self-esteem, helpless, hopeless, guilty or suicidal
RESENTFUL: bitter, angry, irritable
LONELY
COMPLAINS A LOT

Provide supportive visits to give encouragement and maintain confidence

DOES THE PATIENT THINK THE PAIN IS UNDER CONTROL?

YES
Annoying or troublesome, but mostly under control

NO
Pain is miserable, intense, unbearable, frightening, punishing, cruel, vicious

Assess levels of least and worst pain. Encourage judicious use of analgesics when necessary. Identify and encourage avoidance of trigger factors. Encourage, provide, teach, alternative active pain-controlling strategies for patient's own use. Monitor pain-relieving and iatrogenic effects of all drugs.

DOES THE PATIENT FEEL WELL INFORMED ABOUT THE ILLNESS OR PAINFUL CONDITION?

YES
Fully informed or unconcerned

NO
Wishes to know results of tests, cause or potential outcome of present condition

Provide information and feedback.
Involve patient in assessing and monitoring progress.
Refer to GP for information where necessary.
Put in touch with self-help groups.

DOES THE PATIENT FEEL OCCUPIED?

YES
Involved in self-care, social or recreational activities

NO
Feels useless, little or nothing to do

Encourage carers to involve patient in self-care and household activities.
Encourage involvement in social and recreational activities, rather than passive pastimes.
Refer to occupational therapist for aids to independence and advice regarding skills training.

DOES THE PATIENT FEEL DISSATISFIED WITH PAST LIFE OR HAVE SUBSTANTIAL REGRETS?

NO
Feels fulfilled, satisfied

YES
Feels bitter, unfulfilled

Talk about the regrets with patient.
Use a counselling approach and guide towards a more positive assessment of the past, if possible.
Use a religious perspective where appropriate.
Understand the past impact of previous disappointments and be sympathetic.

DOES THE PATIENT HAVE ANY OTHER PROBLEMS TO COPE WITH?

NO
Would be relatively trouble-free without pain

YES
Loss or illness of close relative or friend
Financial or domestic problems

Provide practical help with practical problems, using referrals where necessary (e.g. regarding financial difficulties).
Provide social support during periods of adjustment and gradually encourage alternative active interests.

ARE THERE ANY OTHER POSSIBLE REASONS FOR NEGATIVE FEELINGS, E.G. DEATH ANXIETY, CONCERN ABOUT THE FUTURE, DRUGS, ALCOHOL?

Manage as appropriate

Figure 5.1 The nursing management of elderly patients with pain, in the community. (From Walker *et al.*, 1990, with permission.)

Acceptance of patients' statements

It may be that some patients do not spontaneously verbalize pain. When a patient does, it is important that his report of pain is accepted. Very occasionally a nurse may care for a 'malingerer' but generally speaking, side effects of medication are unwanted and malingerers are few. Accepting and believing statements and reports of pain may rule out the possibility of a patient suffering unnecessarily.

Many people who suffer chronic pain learn to control the expression of their pain and it would be a mistake not to believe such people on occasions when they report pain.

DIFFICULTIES IN ASSESSING PAIN

In one study, nurses were asked to describe one patient situation in which it was difficult to assess pain and one in which it was easy. In general, nurses reported that physiological signs and behaviours were easier to note than verbal reports from the patient. Nurses did not rely so much on the patient's own reports of pain, even though the most reliable indicator of how much pain a person is experiencing is his own verbal subjective report (Jacox, 1979). However, this does not mean that subjective reports are the only ways of assessing pain. We must begin with the recognition that pain is a subjective phenomenon and include the many factors influencing pain in our evaluation.

Misconceptions that may hamper the assessment of pain

The amount of tissue damage is not an accurate predictor of the intensity and duration of pain that a patient may suffer. Sometimes staff may think that patients undergoing similar surgical operations will experience the same intensity and/or duration of pain. The gate control theory of pain proposed by Melzack and Wall (1965) suggested that pain perception may be altered by cerebral influences (see Chapter 7 for further update on this). Past experiences, anxiety level and the context of the trauma may therefore influence a person's response to pain.

A study of wounded soldiers in the Second World War, which is frequently cited in the literature, showed that only 25% of badly injured men complained of pain or requested analgesia, whereas in a group of male civilians undergoing surgery, 80% required analgesia although their tissue damage was similar to that of the soldiers. The soldiers may have seen their wounds as a way of releasing them from duty at the front line and, because they sustained their injuries in a heroic context, they experienced less pain than the civilians who saw surgery as an interruption of their daily lives (Beecher, 1956). A more recent study of patients who underwent appendicectomy in Lebanon following the war in 1975–76 showed that these patients required less analgesia postoperatively than a similar group of patients who underwent similar surgery before the war. The findings implied that patients' perception of pain had changed due to the psychological trauma of war, resulting in patients requiring less analgesia to relieve postoperative pain (Armenian, Chamieh and Barak, 1981).

Routine and tradition

Assessment of pain is further hampered by 'routine' drug rounds in hospitals and/or caring institutions. This routine places constraints on patients who may feel they have to ask for analgesics at that time or accept them if offered. This may be done simply to comply with the ward routine or because a patient knows that the trolley may not be round for another four hours and that he could experience pain before then but would not want to bother a nurse. One patient mentioned that she missed the 6.00 pm trolley because she went to the bathroom. She said:

> I was in agony – I thought the nurses would come back and ask me if I needed painkillers, but they didn't. I think they must have been very busy and I didn't like to ask, so I waited for the night nurses' drug round.

Should patients be expected to gear their pain relief requirements to hospital routines? Good assessment of a patient's pain may reveal that this requirement is either more or less than that which is made available to him from the four-hourly drug trolley round.

Awareness of pain should be a routine item in caring for patients. Edwards (1990) defines the problem of undertreatment of patients as originating in deficiencies in knowledge and skills of staff. In a study to test the effect of education for nurses on postoperative pain of patients, Sofaer (1984) found that greater proportions of patients felt their pain was noticed by staff after a ward based educational programme for staff. The programme highlighted the importance of assessment. It also highlighted the fact that where nurses are exposed to education and encouragement, they respond by helping patients.

INDIVIDUALIZED ASSESSMENT OF PAIN

One argument that has been offered by nurses against individualized assessment of pain is that medical staff often prescribe analgesia 'four hourly' (which may be true even though the duration of action of an analgesic is less than four hours). This does not mean that the nurse must interpret the time of administration necessarily to coincide with routine drug rounds. Indeed, prescribing patterns are becoming more flexible (see Chapter 8). The whole point of pain assessment is that it will reveal whether or not the prescription framework within which a drug is administered is appropriate for an individual patient. If not, the medical staff can be approached and asked if they would be willing to alter the prescription, either to increase or decrease a dose or to increase or decrease the frequency of administration or to prescribe an alternative analgesic with a different intensity or duration of action. One staff nurse using pain assessment commented:

> Each patient's assessments show a different pattern and their individual requirements vary. It is great, we are able to use the assessments to communicate better with the medical staff and they are responding to us.

Having a written record

Because of the individual nature of pain and the variation in its expression, nurses must be prepared to accept some of the responsibility in identifying when a patient is in pain. One way of trying to overcome the difficulties is to use a pain assessment chart (see Figure 5.2). The main advantage of having a written record of pain assessment is that it improves the chance of decreasing suffering by facilitating communication between patients, nurses and medical staff. In one ward where pain assessment had been recorded as part of a research project on the management of postoperative pain, a staff nurse said:

> I feel much more in control of the situation now than before. I am less anxious myself about the possibility of patients suffering unnecessarily. The assessment chart is easy to use and has helped us all to control pain before it gets severe.

Clarke *et al.* (1996) noted that in reviewing charts of patients there was very little in the way of patient self-assessment of pain or any indication of effectiveness of pain interventions. They recommended that a patient self-rating tool be included on the patient's chart alongside vital sign information.

Learning what a patient is experiencing

In order to be effective in her intervention, the nurse must not only be observant, she must be able to examine the factors influencing the patient's pain response and minimize her own prejudices about how pain should be tolerated. There is also the need to find out how the patient usually deals with pain and to enlist his assistance in assessing the pain and in finding ways to relieve it. Above all, a nurse must always be willing to listen to a patient in an empathic way and to accept that only the patient can really know what hurts, when it hurts and how much it hurts.

Assessing the pain with the patient

Pain is assessed *with* the patient and not on the patient. This is a very important point because the patient's own estimate of pain must be used as the basis for treatment. The nurse should not allow her own experiences of pain or her observations in other situations to influence the assessment. As Carroll (1993) points out, there is no reason why a patient cannot complete assessments independently. She notes

PAIN ASSESSMENT CHART
Ward 28

Sheet No. 1

Patient's Name: Mrs MacDonald
Hospital Number: OO 7418

Put a tick in the column which best describes the pain since the last recording

Date	Time	No pain or sleeping	Slight pain	Moderate pain	Severe pain	Pain bad as it could be	Signature of nurse	Site	Comment and/or nursing action	Analgesic given			
										Name	Dose	Route	Time
13.6.97	11.00		✓				P. Smith	abdomen	analgesic given with anti-emetic	Diamorphine	5 mg	I.M.	11.00
	12.10			✓			P. Smith	abdomen	disorientated anti-emetic analgesic given	Diamorphine	5 mg	I.M.	12.15
	13.30	✓					P. Smith	—					
	14.30	✓					P. Smith	—					
	15.30			✓			S/N McCallum	abdomen	analgesic and anti-emetic given	Omnopon	15 mg	I.M.	15.35
	16.30	✓					S/N McCallum	—	appears more settled				
	18.00	✓					S/N McCallum	—					
	20.00			✓			S/N Ford	abdomen	washed + turned, mod. pain following analgesic given	Omnopon	15 mg	I.M.	20.10
	22.00	✓					S/N Ford	—	turned and settled down				
	24.00	✓					S/N T Burns						
14.6.97	01.45		✓				S/N T Burns	abdomen	analgesic given	Omnopon	15 mg	I.M.	01.45

Figure 5.2 A pain assessment chart showing how one patient's pain was assessed and effectively relieved following surgery.

PAIN ASSESSMENT CHART
Ward **8**

Sheet No. _1_
Patient's Name: _Mrs Fraser_
Hospital Number: _274306_

Put a tick in the column which best describes the pain since the last recording

Date	Time	No pain or sleeping	Slight pain	Moderate pain	Severe pain	Pain bad as it could be	Signature of nurse	Site	Comment and/or nursing action	Analgesic given			
										Name	Dose	Route	Time
28.8.97	16.45				✓		P. Jones	abdomen	Required Dr to increase dose (enquired)	Diamorphine	2.5mg	I/M	17.10
	17.40			✓			P. Jones	abdomen					
	19.10		✓				P. Jones	abdomen					
	20.20	✓					P. Jones						
	21.15			✓			P. Jones	abdomen	Required Dr to increase dose (enquired)	Diamorphine	2.5mg	I/M	21.20
	22.00			✓			J. Frost	abdomen					
	23.20			✓			J. Frost	abdomen	analgesia	Diamorphine	2.5mg	I/M	23.25
29.8.97	24.00	✓					J. Frost						
	02.00		✓				M. Freeman	abdomen					
	03.30	✓					M. Freeman						
	04.00						M. Freeman	abdomen	analgesic given	Diamorphine	2.5	I/M	04.30
	04.30	✓					M. Freeman						
	06.00	✓					M. Freeman						

Figure 5.3 A pain assessment chart showing how pain relief was delayed.

that the success of assessment lies in the frequency with which the charts are evaluated by nursing and medical staff.

Figure 5.2 illustrates a pain assessment chart showing how one patient's pain was assessed and relieved effectively following surgery. Figure 5.3 illustrates a chart showing how pain relief was delayed, even though the nurse making the assessment informed the medical staff that analgesia was not effective. This patient experienced considerable suffering.

To elicit descriptions of pain and to assess changes in the nature and severity of pain over time, a pain description chart might be helpful. Patients may be asked to select from a list of adjectives, such as 'mild', 'distressing', 'knifelike', 'throbbing' or 'cramping', those words that best describe the pain. It might also be possible to connect an episode of pain with a bodily function or a time of day and thereby help the patient to find ways of avoiding such pain-inducing situations.

Pain in children

Assessing pain in children may present further difficulties. Many children endure unacceptable pain during their stay in hospital and prevention and management must be improved (Cummings *et al.*, 1996). In a recent report, Zonneveld *et al.* (1997) suggest that children do remember pain accurately and that memory does not fade over a period of a week.

Parents play a role in assessing their children's pain and their attitudes are important (Forward, Brown and McGrath, 1996). The effectiveness of relevant play in preparing children for painful procedures is very important, but words are not reliable in communicating with very young children when trying to assess the location and intensity of pain. Play presents information in a more understandable way and young children readily identify with and project feelings onto a special doll or teddy. A nurse could therefore exploit such play to find out the location of pain. An older child might be able to point to the site of pain on a body chart. The literature on pain management with children has increased hugely in recent years. Interested readers are referred to the following excellent texts on pain and children: McGrath and Unruh, 1987; McGrath, Ritchie and Unruh, 1993; and Carter, 1994.

Use of an analogue scale

Since pain is a subjective experience, it may be useful to provide a patient with a scale on which the extremes of the experience are indicated (Figure 5.4).

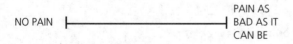

Figure 5.4 A visual analogue scale (after Scott and Huskisson, 1976).

The patient is asked to place a mark on the scale to represent the level of pain at the time. The distance of the mark from the left-hand end of the scale is the pain score. The scale may be used several times during a day. A pain profile (Figure 5.5) may then be constructed to show if treatment has been effective.

Intervals between pain assessments

There are no set rules regarding the time interval between pain assessments for the same patient. It is, however, important that nurses record the administration and subsequent effect of an analgesic or other pain-relieving strategy.

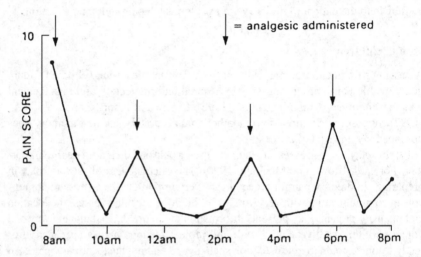

Figure 5.5 A pain profile showing the effect of analgesia on pain score (after Bond, 1979). Arrows indicate the times at which an analgesic was administered.

Circumstances vary from one situation to another. It may be that following surgery, pain assessment would be appropriate every one or two hours for the first two days, with the frequency of assessment being decreased subsequently. It is strongly recommended that the assessment chart is left at the patient's bedside. Since no patient would be left for more than two hours without some member of staff coming to the bedside, the process of pain assessment does not involve extra staff and requires little additional time.

Assessing chronic pain

In assessing chronic pain, a body chart may be helpful to the patient in locating pain. It also provides a means whereby the site of pain can be documented. You can make up a body chart by drawing a simple outline of the front and back views of the body. A patient may then be asked to indicate the site of his pain by marking the chart. Any changes can be noted on subsequent charts and recordings may be made of any action taken to relieve the pain.

Patients who experience chronic pain might find it helpful to have their pain assessed twice daily to check the efficacy of analgesia. For patients who are nursed at home, a home assessment record could be useful in disclosing patterns of pain and facilitating adjustments in therapy by the doctor.

Sometimes the McGill Pain Questionnaire can be a useful tool. It can be used for both acute and chronic pain assessment (see Melzack and Wall, 1996). One advantage is that it does consider the character of the pain. It is used mostly in research settings and in pain centres in the USA. A major disadvantage is that it can take up to 20 minutes to complete (see Carroll (1993) for further information and replication of a short version of the McGill Pain Questionnaire).

Comfort measures

Repositioning, smoothing the bed and offering a warm drink can help a patient to relax. Although these measures may not relieve severe pain, they may sometimes relieve discomfort or mild pain, making more potent therapies unnecessary. The following anecdote illustrates this point. A patient returned from the operating theatre following a transurethral prostatectomy. He reported pain and an opioid analgesic was administered. The cause of the pain was not investigated. He remained restless and agitated and looked unwell. The staff nurse noticed that the urethral catheter was not draining, so she performed a bladder washout. A litre of fluid was removed. The patient settled, slept well and his colour returned to normal. The nurse later commented that in this instance an obvious cause for the pain had been a full bladder and that it had served as a good learning experience, where an analgesic had not been required and should not have been given prior to other measures being taken.

PATIENTS' VIEWS

The experience of pain has been described by one author as including both the stimulus and response to that stimulus and she has analysed the 'experience' of patients in terms of 'suffering' (Copp, 1974). In the course of her research she asked patients what nurses and doctors could do about pain. Patients suggested that there is nothing more important than talking to patients about pain and that nurses should be prompt and try to understand. Nurses, they suggested, should also stop telling people they do not have pain when they actually do and not try to feel for people when they can't know if patients have pain or not. Having confidence can help relieve the pain; if nurses had more confidence patients would too. Patients also felt that nurses should not assume that medication helps. Copp also examined how nurses appear to patients in response to a request for pain relief. A patient may see the nurse as acting in a variety of roles:

- *a controller* – relieving or denying relief;
- *a communicator* – passing on, validating and interpreting the bid for pain reduction;
- *a judge* – deciding if pain is reasonable, timely and expected in terms of quality and quantity;
- *an avoider* – refusing to report that medication does not bring relief;
- *an empathizer* – letting the patient have his own experience; an authentic empathizer 'knows' and 'has experiences'; a pseudoempathizer responds by describing her own experience to obtain feelings of credit or to rob the patient of attention;
- *a barterer* – giving relief in return for good patient behaviour.

Nurses' awareness of how their own behaviour might affect a patient's response to pain and its assessment has further implications. For example, if a nurse acts in a judgemental way, relief may be given to the patient in order to salve the nurse's conscience and not because the nurse herself really believes in what the patient is saying.

PREREQUISITES FOR NURSES ASSESSING PAIN

An awareness of ethical codes in relation to patient rights is a first step. A background knowledge of the theoretical concepts involved in the complex phenomenon of pain is the next. Displaying acceptance of individual patients' differences in pain tolerance and coping patterns are also basic prerequisites for any nurse who wishes to be effective in relieving pain. Working as part of a multidisciplinary team is so important. With real collaboration, everybody can benefit.

References

Allcock, N. (1996) Factors affecting the assessment of postoperative pain: a literature review. *Journal of Advanced Nursing*, **24**, 1144–51.

Armenian, H. K., Chamieh, M. A. and Barak, A. (1981) Influences of war-time stress and psychosocial factors in Lebanon on analgesic requirements for post-operative pain. *Social Science and Medicine*, **151**, 63–6.

Beecher, H. K. (1956) Relationship of significance of wound to pain experienced. *Journal of the American Medical Association*, **161**, 1609–13.

Bond, M. R. (1979) *Pain: Its Nature, Analysis and Treatment*, Churchill Livingstone, Edinburgh.

Camp, L. and O'Sullivan, P. (1987) Comparison of medical, surgical and oncology patients' descriptions of pain and nurses' documentation of pain assessments. *Journal of Advanced Nursing*, **12**(5), 593-8.

Carroll, D. (1993) Pain assessment, in *Pain Management and Nursing Care*, (eds D. Carroll and D. Bewsher), Butterworth-Heinemann, Oxford.

Carter, B (1994) *Child and Infant Pain*, Chapman and Hall, London.

Choiniere, M., Melzack, R., Girard, N., Rondeau, J. and Paquin, M. (1990) Comparisons between patients' and nurses' assessment of pain and medication in severe burn injuries. *Pain*, **40**, 143-52.

Clarke, E. B., French, B., Bilodeau, M.I. *et al.* (1996) Pain management knowledge, attitudes and clinical practice: the impact of nurses' characteristics and education. *Journal of Pain and Symptom Management*, **11**(1), 18–31

Cohen, F. (1980) Postsurgical pain relief: patients' status and nurses' medication choices. *Pain*, **9**, 265–74.

Copp, L. A. (1974) The spectrum of suffering. *American Journal of Nursing*, **74**, 491–5.

Cummings, E. A., Reid, G. J., Finley, G. A., McGrath P. J. and Ritchie, J. A. (1996) Prevalence and source of pain in pediatric inpatients. *Pain*, **68**, 25–31.

Dufault, M., Bielechi, C., Collins, E. and Willey, C. (1995) Changing nurses' pain assessment practice: a collaborative research utilization approach. *Journal of Advanced Nursing*, **21**, 634–45.

Edwards, W. T. (1990) Optimizing opioid treatment of postoperative pain. *Journal of Pain and Symptom Management*, **5** (Supp 1), S24–36.

Ferrell, B. (1991) Pain management as a quality care outcome. *Journal of Nursing Quality Assurance*, **5**, 2.

Forward, S. P., Brown, T. L. and McGrath P. J. (1996) Mothers' attitudes and behaviour toward medicating children's pain. *Pain*, **67**, 469–74.

Gagliese, L. and Melzack, R. (1997) Chronic pain in elderly people. *Pain*, **70**(1), 3–14.

Hardy, L. K. (1990) The path to nursing knowledge–personal reflections. *Nurse Education Today*, **10**, 325–32.

Harrison, A. (1991) Assessing patients' pain: identifying reasons for error. *Journal of Advanced Nursing*, **16**, 1018–25.

Jacox, A. K. (1979) Assessing pain. *American Journal of Nursing*, **79**, 895–900.

Lander, J. (1990) Clinical judgement in pain management. *Pain*, **42**(1), 15–22.

Mackintosh, C. (1994) Do nurses provide adequate post-operative pain relief? *British Journal of Nursing*, **3**(7), 15–18.

Marks, R. M. and Sachar, E. J. (1973) Undertreatment of medical inpatients with narcotic analgesics. *Annals of Internal Medicine*, **78**, 173-81.

McCaffery, M. (1983) *Nursing the Patient in Pain*, Harper and Row, London.

McGrath, P. J. and Unruh, A. M. (1987) *Pain in Children and Adolescents, Vol. 1, Pain Research and Clinical Management*, Elsevier, Amsterdam.

McGrath, P. J., Ritchie, J. A. and Unruh, A. M. (1993) Paediatric pain, in *Pain Management and Nursing Care*, (eds D. Carroll and D. Bowsher), Butterworth-Heinemann, Oxford.

Melzack, R. and Wall, P. D. (1965) Pain mechanisms: a new theory. *Science*, **150**, 971–9.

Melzack, R and Wall, P.D. (1996) *The Challenge of Pain*, Penguin Books, London.

Scott, J. and Huskisson, E. C. (1976) Graphic representation of pain. *Pain*, **2**, 175–84.

Seers, K. (1989) Patients' perceptions of acute pain, in *Directions in Nursing Research: Ten Years of Progress at London University*, (eds J. Wilson Barnett and S. Robinson), Scutari, London, pp. 107–116.

Sofaer, B. (1984) The effect of focused education for nursing teams on postoperative pain of patients. Unpublished PhD thesis, University of Edinburgh.

Tanabe, P. (1995) Recognising pain as a component of the primary assessment. Adding D for discomfort to the ABC's. *Journal of Emergency Nursing*, **21**(4), 299–304.

Walker, J. (1993) Pain in the elderly, in *Pain Management and Nursing Care*, (eds D. Carroll and D. Bowsher), Butterworth-Heinemann, Oxford.

Walker, J. M., Akinsanya, J. A., Davis, B. D. and Marcer, D. (1990) The nursing management of elderly patients with pain in the community: study and recommendations. *Journal of Advanced Nursing*, **15**, 1154–61.

Weiner, D., Pieper, C., McConnell, E., Martinez, S. and Keefe, F. (1996) Pain measurement in elders with chronic low back pain: traditional and alternative approaches. *Pain*, **67**(2 &3), 461–7.

Weis, O. F., Sriwatanakul, K., Alloza, J. L., Weintraub, M. and Lasagna, L. (1983) Attitudes of patients, housestaff and nurses towards postoperative analgesic care. *Anaesthesia and Analgesia*, **62**, 72–4.

Zonneveld, L. N. L., McGrath, P. J., Reid, G. J. and Sorbi, M. J. (1997) Accuracy of children's pain memories. *Pain*, **71**(3), 297–302.

'The cholecystectomy in bed 21' 6

Reflect on how skilfully and gently your colic makes you lose your taste for life and detaches you from the world – not compelling you by some tyrannous subjection as do so many other afflictions found in old men which keep them continually fettered to weakness and unremittingly in pain but with intermittent warnings and counsels interspersed with long periods of respite, as if to give you the means to meditate on its lesson and to go over it again at leisure. And so as to give you the means to make a sound judgement and to be resolved like a sensible man, it shows you the state of the whole human condition, both good and bad, shows you during one single day, a life at times full of great joy, at times unbearable. Although you may not throw your arms about Death's neck, you do, once a month, shake her by the hand.

Michel [de] Montaigne

When it was decided to write a third edition of this book this chapter was not planned. Things came to a temporary halt after writing Chapter 5 as a result of several attacks of biliary colic. The result is a personal account of those experiences and of surgery. I don't know if fate was a good or bad thing, but it taught me something about horrendous pain and about not being in control. Now I am able to relate the experiences to you as a patient. There was a real dilemma about the placement of this chapter. After consultation with the publisher and colleagues, it was decided it was not appropriate to place it at the beginning nor at the end of the book. So we decided to leave it here. After all, in the context of time, it is quite appropriate, because the events related here happened just after I had finished writing Chapter 5.

There is a departure in style in this chapter. It was necessary to 'change gear' and to present it in the first person. What follows is my 'story' as it happened.

BACKGROUND AND HISTORY

One night in the middle of December 1996 I awoke with pain the like of which I had never experienced in my life. I crawled to the bathroom and en route unlocked the front door. I phoned a neighbour and asked for help. The next couple of hours were spent writhing, sweating, shaking, vomiting and begging the neighbour for a doctor. My neighbour phoned the emergency services three times but the doctor on call was attending to a heart attack victim and was unavailable. By the time the doctor phoned me back the pain had vanished and I went off to sleep. I thought it must have been a 'one off' attack of something. My mind was occupied with other problems and I forgot about the event.

A couple of weeks later, on Christmas Day, following lunch with my family (which included roast duck and Christmas pudding) the same thing happened but the attack was of shorter duration and, feeling perfectly well the following day, I drove 150 miles home. I didn't think about these attacks at all until 3rd January 1997 when, following a light lunch, yet again the very same thing happened. For the next two days I felt horrible. I felt very nauseous, I had a distended abdomen, a slight pyrexia and I felt very tired. Two days later I consulted my GP, who diagnosed cholecystitis, started me on an antibiotic (Augmentin), suggested a low fat diet, took blood for liver function tests and arranged an ultrasound examination of the gallbladder. I mentioned to him that I wasn't overly fond of milky foods.

I returned to see the GP five days later, still feeling unwell. Liver function tests were normal. He recommended a continuation of the antibiotic. I stayed on a low (actually a 'no') fat diet and underwent an ultrasound examination on 20th January. The radiologist told me the gallbladder was 'packed with calculi' and I wasn't to eat as much as a 'molecule of fat'. A repeat liver function test again showed normal results. Referral was made to a surgeon but, based on clinical need at the time, no appointment was available until the beginning of March (almost two months later). Beds were very much at a premium and understandably priority had to be given to patients who had cancer.

I suffered another attack a few days later. A neighbour who witnessed it thought it revealing that although I was able to advise others on control of pain, I became 'a hostage to it in same way as anyone else would'. My neighbour told me several weeks later: 'You would say "I'll give it 15 minutes then I will call a doctor" and a minute later you would look at the clock and say "is it only a minute?".'

It was decided to refer me to another surgeon who saw me at the end of January and confirmed that surgery was required. An open cholecystectomy was planned. Following an experiment with poached fish I experienced yet another attack. I was offered a bed for surgery to take place on 20th February (due to a cancellation), but with the warning that my surgery might be cancelled if no beds were available because of emergencies.

'CLERKING IN'

The system for clerking in patients was excellent not only in terms of efficiency but also from the point of view of humaneness. Two days prior to admission, I was seen in outpatients by a member of the surgical team. Blood and other tests were carried out and I was given information about the procedures. There was also an opportunity to ask questions of the surgeon. This was helpful. I expressed anxiety about having an anaesthetic (I had had a bad experience some 20 years ago with an anaesthetic drug). I wasn't anxious about the surgery. I didn't feel that was my worry. Neither was I worried about postoperative pain – 'Anyone who is afraid of suffering suffers already of being afraid' (Montaigne).

I looked forward to being able to eat normal foods. With the exception of the couple of experiments I had stuck rigidly to eating only pulses, fruit and vegetables for several weeks.

During the period since the first attack of biliary colic, I had managed (just) to keep my head above water. Some days I was less well than others but for the most part I managed to maintain my teaching commitments and my counselling sessions with patients who suffered chronic pain. I did, however, have a worry which took my attention away from myself. One of my children was awaiting neurosurgery for removal of a tumour from his frontal bone (which later proved to be benign). I felt it was important for me to be able to cope well with my own surgery and to rehabilitate myself as soon as possible so that I would be available to offer support to him.

Having been clerked in, I felt a sense of proportion about the impending hospitalization. However, the events of the following day (the day before admission), Tuesday 18th February, will remain in my memory for a while.

> They see you sweating under the strain, turning pale, flushing, trembling, sicking up everything ... suffering curious spasms and convulsions, sometimes shedding huge tears from your eyes ... (Montaigne)

I didn't feel well in the morning, but I couldn't pinpoint why. I did some counselling with a patient, had a light lunch of fruit and vegetables and set off to drive about 20 miles to teach students.

Just before arrival I felt pain coming on. I reached the car park and vomited and vomited. The pain was horrendous. I cannot describe it. A student and a colleague tried to support me for the next hour and 40 minutes while I writhed, wept, shook, whispered, banged my fists on the floor and on the walls. I held on to anything or anybody and was held. I felt ill. I felt pale. I felt old. I felt as if I was going to die. I vomited many times. I went to the toilet and came back from the toilet, took off my skirt and loosened my bra. Nothing helped. No amount of holding, writhing, praying or crying helped. Sitting, lying or standing made no difference whatsoever. The pain was relentless. A colleague wanted to call an ambulance. I refused. The pain was too severe to go anywhere and especially to a hospital which was not the one where surgery had been arranged for the following day. 'It will end,' I said. And of course it did. And I felt fine. I took an analgesic which stayed down, had a drink of water and after about an hour of being pain free started driving home escorted by three of the students.

About 15 minutes from home the pain started again and I was unable to continue. One of the students drove me home and summoned the GP, who visited and agreed that I should be admitted as planned the following day. I slept well but the following morning yet again had another encounter with biliary colic. The doctor wanted to send me to hospital by ambulance but I was in too much pain to go anywhere and I did not want to face the drama of going into an accident and emergency department. I waited until the pain eased a bit, confirmed with the hospital that there was indeed a bed for me and went in a colleague's car to the hospital. I mention this because in other places in the book, I discuss the effect of family values and culture on individual expressions of pain and pain behaviour. During the days preceding my admission, I kept at the back of my mind some conversations I had had with my late grandmother. She had lived through two world wars. She would *not* have gone to hospital in an ambulance!

THE ADMISSION

It has been suggested (in this book and in many other nursing and medical texts) that putting the patient at ease by giving an explanation of what is going to happen will help prevent postoperative problems and may, in some personalities, reduce pain following surgery.

My admission (both medical and nursing) was absolutely excellent. The staff were sensitive and I was listened to and spoken to as an equal. In view of the two attacks just prior to my admission, blood was again taken for liver function tests. The nurse who carried out the 'nursing assessment' knew something about human beings. (She had a wholesomeness about her and a soft Irish sincerity which were endearing.) Her admission questions and nursing assessment were entirely appropriate and carried out with sensitivity and in a sensible manner. I really felt reassured by her and also by a note from the anaesthetist to say that he would see me early the following morning.

I felt ill but reasonably calm and I slept well. I was optimistic about the surgery and the outcome.

The anaesthetist arrived as promised the next morning. He asked me what I 'wanted' and when I replied that I would like to have an epidural postoperatively if possible, he said, 'I usually do that anyway!' I also asked not to be catheterized unless absolutely necessary. He seemed to think that was a reasonable request.

My premedication worked satisfactorily. Just before departure for theatre, the surgeon came to the ward and told me that as my liver function tests done the previous day were not normal, it would be necessary to do 'an old fashioned cholecystectomy and an on-table cholangiogram'. I was a little concerned that I might end up with a 'T' tube but I accepted that if it was necessary then that was what would happen. The fact that the surgeon took the trouble to tell me was appreciated. I was somewhat upset, however, to be told by a staff nurse just before I went to theatre that if I needed a nasogastric tube when I returned to the ward then they would 'put one down'!

There was a short, bumpy and somewhat cold ride and then I was in theatre. A quick 'scratch' in the back of my hand and no time to say goodbye or hello! It was just before 2.00 pm.

THE POSTOPERATIVE EXPERIENCE

The next thing I remember was seeing a nurse's head peeping through the curtains at the bottom of my bed: 'Beatrice, it is all over, your blood pressure is low. I am offering you a catheter'. I remember replying 'No thank you'. Then I recall my eldest daughter kissing me on the right cheek and saying 'Ima (Hebrew for Mother), I'll be back to see you in the morning.' It was around 7.30 pm and I was now back in the ward. I don't remember a thing about the recovery room.

It is no exaggeration to say that the first postoperative night was very difficult indeed. I had an epidural (bupivacaine 0.15%) running at 5 ml per hour. I was getting partial relief but still experiencing quite a bit of pain. This was made worse by the fact that I had difficulty passing urine and I needed to be propped up. But the staff didn't prop me up and my body was at an angle of about 30°. I was uncomfortable. Adding to my difficulty was the fact that I was attached to nasal oxygen, an intravenous infusion, the epidural, a drain from the wound, a blood pressure cuff and pulse oximeter machine. There wasn't much room for manoeuvre and the staff were too busy to stay with me while I was on the bedpan. I became distressed with the situation.

I was in severe pain around 1.00 am. I discovered later that the staff nurse had turned off the epidural. I asked for Omnopon which I had been written up for. The nurse refused. 'I am reluctant to give it to you.' We argued.

Later, the nurse adjusted the epidural and I persuaded her to increase the infusion to 7 ml per hour (recorded as 2.00 am). By 3.00 am I managed to pass urine. At 5.00 am I asked for the Omnopon but my request was again refused. We had another 'discussion'. It was, I recall, a little heated. I said 'Nobody need suffer postoperative pain like this'. Tersely, she responded, 'You only get pain relief in an ideal world, I have read your book, I can understand you don't like not being in control' (read the book, I thought to myself, but missed the point!). 'Cholecystectomy is a painful operation and you must expect to have pain. I'll change your sheet.' She changed the top sheet. (A few months later, when I told this story to a colleague, she said that the clean sheet probably cost more than giving pain relief!) 'But I am written up for Omnopon,' I said pleadingly. 'I can't give it without checking,' she said. 'Well, check then', I replied. 'I am too busy, we have a lot to do, there are nine post-op patients'. With a sense of resignation, I said 'It will go in Chapter 6'.

I had a clean top sheet and an awful lot of pain. In my mind's eye I could see the expression on the face of the patient whose narrative appears in Chapter 1 as she said to me, 'I thought they (the staff) are there to look after you'.

There is ample evidence to show that postoperative pain can and should be relieved. I was in too much pain to think of 'evidence' – I just wanted relief. It hurt to move. It hurt to cough. It hurt to cry. I closed my eyes. I felt deserted and betrayed. And even my own sense of soul left me. I felt a huge sense of failure.

At 7.45 am on the morning following surgery a small figure in blue appeared and held my left hand between hers. I shall never forget those moments. It was my colleague to whom this book is dedicated. 'What a state you are in,' she exclaimed. She set to work and restored my sense of being and dignity. She helped me wash, tidied me up, helped me into some clean clothes. She noticed that the epidural burette was completely empty (hardly any wonder I was in pain). She filled it up and within minutes I began to feel relief. Over lunch a month later, she told me that when she arrived 'Your eyes were in horror with pain'.

At 9.10 am, the anaesthetist arrived. He said 'You are unhappy'. The epidural infusion was increased to 10 ml per hour. He prescribed diclofenac (Voltarol) PR 100 mg stat to be followed by 50 mg eight-hourly. 'It will work like a treat.' And it did. For the rest of that day I had marvellous pain control. I was able to get in and out of bed without pain. The nurses encouraged me. But coughing was hell! The physiotherapist was sympathetic and I deep-breathed and huffed as instructed. I was terrified of getting a chest infection (echoes of Chapter 1).

The day following surgery passed without much pain except when I tried to cough. A young doctor doing a ward round inspected the IV cannula and pulled back the adhesive holding it in place. I yelped 'ouch', to which he responded in a rather sergeant-majorish voice, 'Just relax'.

The combination of Voltarol and the epidural gave me good analgesia although after about seven hours I was beginning to need the Voltarol again. The IV and drain were removed and mobility was easier. The second postoperative night was not too bad. I slept for two three-hour periods until 4.00 am. I was in pain then but was not 'due' the Voltarol until 6.00 am. I was offered Omnopon, this time by a very kindly night nurse, but I declined because I wanted to avoid the side effects. So I hung on and welcomed the early morning 6.00 am dose of Voltarol.

It was now Saturday 22nd February. I felt quite tired. I was interested to hear from the nurses that they planned to take down the epidural. The dose was reduced to 7 ml per hour but at 5.00 pm it was obvious that I wasn't coping well. At about 8.00 pm the staff nurse called the on-call anaesthetist for advice. He came to see me. He evaluated the situation and suggested that the epidural remain up for the night. The top bag needed replacing so he replaced it with the same as before (0.15% bupivacaine). He increased the dose back to 10 ml per hour.

That night was not brilliant. I felt I had to clear my chest. (In the past year I had had two chest infections and I didn't want another one.) I slept on and off but needed help to hold my ribs while I coughed on a couple of occasions. A young student nurse helped me.

On the third postoperative day, the enrolled nurse 'in charge' of the bay where my bed was, said, 'This is coming down' (the epidural). Accordingly, the amount per hour was reduced. I was desperate anyway to get up and have a shower. I wasn't in constant pain but when I moved it was sharp around the wound site. I felt a bit low. (A colleague told me several weeks later that when she visited that day I appeared 'powerless' and had a 'low mood'.) The staff wanted to take down the epidural but then they decided that they didn't have time. Although I would have liked to have had a shower before my visitors arrived, I waited until the beginning of a new shift before the epidural was removed. The dose of Voltarol didn't give me enough pain relief and when the epidural finally was removed at 3.15 pm I did begin to feel very uncomfortable. By 5.00 pm I was in a lot of pain but 'not due' for a further dose of Voltarol until 10.00 pm. At 9.00 pm, I was distressed and the on-call anaesthetist came to see me. He ordered 100 mg of Voltarol PR stat and two sleeping pills. He also told me that he thought the epidural had come down too soon.

I slept until about 3.30 am when I got up and walked up and down the ward in pain. There were two pains, one in my scapula similar to that which I had experienced before surgery and another, central abdominal pain. At 6.00 am, I had a dose of Voltarol. During the day pain continued on and off, more on than off. The staff nurse in charge of the ward was concerned and sympathetic and phoned a doctor for advice. Buscopan two tablets was tried in the afternoon with no effect and later on I had two paracetamol and a Gaviscon tablet which I found in my handbag. These seemed to be effective and I suspected I had some gastric irritation. I had had very little to eat for five days and quite a lot of non-steroidal analgesics both before and following surgery. These can cause gastric irritation.

HOME

In the evening of the fourth postoperative day I was discharged home. It was pouring with rain as a colleague drove me home but the shining streets and the reflection of the lights were nothing in comparison to the shine I felt in my heart to be out of hospital. I was delighted to be again in my own environment. It seemed so quiet and peaceful. I was cared for exceptionally well by a young colleague that night but in the early hours I had severe central abdominal pain. This was relieved by eating some boiled rice followed by Gaviscon. The following morning I was prescribed Aspav (aspirin and papaveretum) and Zantac 300 mg six-hourly. I continued this regime for 24 hours and decreased the doses for another 24 hours. Except for a couple of paracetamol on another occasion, I had no more analgesics. The wound area remained tender but I was very mobile and agile. Mostly this tenderness was due to the siting of the incision which was just below my waistline. Coughing and sneezing caused a bit of pain but otherwise I made excellent progress.

PLEASANT FEELINGS AND PAIN

> I so order my soul that it can contemplate both pain and pleasure with eyes equally restrained ... doing so with eyes equally steady ... (Montaigne)

From a philosophical standpoint it is interesting (and fun) to think about the complexities of life and how they were viewed in the 16th century. From a humanitarian perspective and a purely practical point of view in the 20th century, when technology and knowledge have advanced to a point where suffering can be avoided, it is fair to say that the opposite of pain is not pleasure, but 'no pain'!

However, Montaigne wrote:

> Plato couples pain and pleasure together and wants it to be the duty of fortitude to fight the same fight against pain and against the seductive fascination of immoderate pleasure.

Two weeks to the day since I had surgery, it is a glorious spring day. I am having no difficulty with the 'seductive fascination' of listening to Mozart piano sonatas or of seeing the yellow daffodils as they begin to peep through in the garden. I have no difficulty waking up to the sound of birdsong. And I have no difficulty whatsoever enjoying the texture and taste of an avocado pear. Although I am experiencing nightmares (which seem to have to do with the first postoperative night), enjoyment and appreciation of simple things in life seem to have increased.

SPECIAL PEOPLE

I wish to thank my children and friends for their encouragement through surgery. The consultants (surgeon and anaesthetist) and my GP all helped me hugely.

There are two people, though, for whom I have special words of gratitude. The first is a student nurse (whose name I do not know), who found me in tears with pain, trying to cough. She literally leapt on the bed, put her arms around me and said 'Pleeeeeze don't cry!' I was so taken aback I pulled myself together. She placed her hands on my ribs and helped me to cough. Just as she was about to leave to attend to another patient, she popped her head through the curtains rather shyly and said, 'I remember your lectures on pain from two years ago'.

The other person (for whom words are totally inadequate) is my colleague Carroll Siu. When, on the first postoperative morning she appeared (as I described earlier), she took my hand between her hands. I was feeling as if humanity and myself had deserted me and she introduced integrity and decorum into the situation. She restored balance where there had been imbalance. By the time my children visited they knew their mother was coping okay.

A few weeks later I found a lovely piece of music and reading the libretto I came across the following words:

Those are unknown mysteries
the eternal keeps to himself.
Down upon every heart,
that lodges grievous pain,
he sends one of his clement rays.

Antonio Caldara

And finally, more words from Montaigne:

We must learn to suffer whatever we cannot avoid. Our life is composed, like the harmony of the world, of discords as well as of different tones, sweet and harsh, sharp and flat, soft and loud. If a musician liked only some of them, what could he sing? He has got to know how to use all of them and blend them together. So too must we with good and ill, which are of one substance with our life. Without such blending our being cannot be: one category is no less necessary than the other.

The writings of Montaigne get a bit boring at times, but he experienced pain and he wrote about it vividly so I think the above quotation makes a fitting end to this chapter.

I leave you, in the context of the rest of the book, to draw your own conclusions.

References

Caldara, A. (c.1700) *Maddalena ai piedi di Cristo*, Schola Cantorum Basiliensis, Harmonia Mundi (1996).

(de) Montaigne, M. (1991) 13, On experience, in *The Complete Essays* (trans M. A. Screech), Penguin Classics, Harmondsworth.

7 | The science of pain: an update

Jackie Bentley

It has long been realized that recognizing and responding to pain requires the activity of the peripheral and central nervous system. Peripheral systems are responsible for the detection of injury (nociception) and the transmission of impulses generated to the spinal cord. The spinal cord has been viewed as a 'relay system' transferring incoming information from the peripheries to centres in the brain, where the information can then be processed and the appropriate response generated to remove the individual from harm. Although essentially not inaccurate, this highly simplistic view belies the true complexities of the physiological processes involved and, perhaps more importantly, fails to account for the clinical experience of pain, especially chronic pain syndromes, which nurses must help to manage.

In 1965 Melzack and Wall first published an account of a new theory of pain which they called the 'gate control theory' (see Figure 7.1). Unlike previous theories, especially the specificity theory, this theory tried to account for the many situations when the intensity of the noxious stimuli and pain perceived by the individual are poorly related. Considerable efforts have been made in recent years to provide a physiological basis for the gate control theory and ultimately to unravel the mysteries surrounding pain perception. The account given here is a brief summary of our current understanding of pain, generated by a wealth of recent research findings. Those seeking greater detail should refer to Melzack and Wall's own most recent work *The Challenge of Pain* (1996) and chapters by Devor, Dickenson and Wall in Campbell (1996), which have proved invaluable in writing this chapter. Reviewing a chapter on the nervous system in an anatomy and physiology textbook might also improve an understanding of the physiology of pain.

THE GATE CONTROL THEORY

The gate control theory views pain perception as a series of stages (Figure 7.1). The first stage involves the transmission of noxious stimuli by small diameter peripheral nerve fibres (C and A-delta fibres) to 'transmission cells' in the dorsal horn of the spinal cord. The transmission cells convey impulses to other areas of the spinal cord (e.g. to generate reflex responses) and to the brain. Their activity is central to the experience of pain. Once the transmission cells are stimulated, their activity is maintained for an extended period, possibly by the activity of 'excitatory interneurones', a process referred to as 'wind up' (Dickenson, 1996).

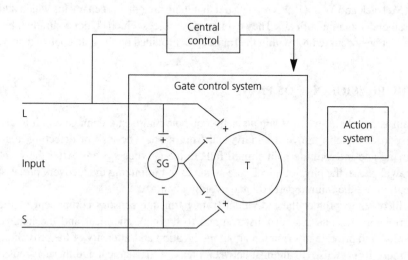

Figure 7.1 Schematic diagram of the gate control theory of pain mechanisms. L, large diameter fibres: S, small diameter fibres. The fibres project to the substantia gelatinosa (SG) and first central transmission cells (T). The inhibitory effect exerted by SG on the afferent fibre terminals is increased by activity in L fibres and decreased by activity in S fibres. The central control trigger is represented by a line running from the large-fibre system to the central control mechanisms: these mechanisms, in turn, project back to the gate control system. The T cells project to the entry cells of the action system. +, excitation: -, inhibition. (From Melzack and Wall, 1965, p. 975.)

Transmission across the synapse relies on chemical neurotransmitters and as such is a process which can be both facilitated or inhibited. Input from large diameter fibres can have either effect on transmitter cells. The small, densely packed area of cells referred to as the substantia gelatinosa contains inhibitory and excitatory interneurones which dampen or amplify output from the transmission cells. The inhibitory effect of these cells is increased by transmission cell stimulation by large diameter fibres (fibres which relay information about touch) and reduced by the small diameter fibres responsible for pain impulses. This implies that inhibitory mechanisms have to be overridden before pain impulses can progress. This is the basis of the 'gating' mechanism advocated by the theory.

The final feature of the gate control theory relates to the influence which the brain has on sensory impulses travelling to the brain from the spinal cord. It is hypothesized that impulses descending from the brain influence inhibitory interneurones. This 'descending inhibitory control' can in turn be influenced by impulses ascending the spinal cord. Thus, impulses from the brain and presumably other areas of the spinal cord (indirectly) can be responsible for operating the 'gate' and so influence the experience of pain.

Melzack and Wall (1996) recognized that there are other mechanisms which add to an understanding of pain. They explained processes which do not contradict, but cannot be accounted for within the framework provided by the gate control theory.

THE PHYSIOLOGY OF PAIN

Pain is beneficial when it signals actual or potential tissue damage and initiates responses which remove the individual from harm. The task of detecting, conveying and interpreting pain stimuli falls to the nervous system. After the withdrawal phase, the physiological state switches to optimizing the recovery process, i.e. holding the injured part still and avoiding contact.

In order to protect the individual from harm, the sensory component of the peripheral nervous system must respond to thermal, chemical and mechanical energy and provide information about the location and intensity of the provoking stimuli. It must also distinguish between pleasant mechanical and thermal sensations and those which are noxious. Although there is a growing view that it is artificial to assume that pain begins with peripheral stimuli (as this approach fails to take into consideration pre-existing factors such as past experience and anxiety, which the gate control theory assumes influence our interpretation of incoming stimuli; Wall, 1996), this is chosen as the starting point for the current account.

PERIPHERAL EVENTS IN NOCICEPTION

Receptors to painful stimuli are found in abundance in skin, muscle, tendon, the articular surfaces and periosteum of bone and in arterial walls and abdominal organs. They are present but less prolific in other deep tissue structures. Although some nerve fibres end in specialized sensory corpuscles, those responsible for the detection of painful stimuli end in extensively branched fibres which overlap to infiltrate the receptive field of neighbouring receptors. This tangle of fibres ensures that the stimulation of one area of tissue results in the stimulation of more than one receptor.

Classically, sensory nerve fibres have been categorized in three groups:

1. A-beta fibres are large in diameter and myelinated. They transmit impulses at speeds of 30–100 m/s and are described as 'low threshold fibres' because minimal stimulation is required to generate an impulse. They respond to light touch.

2. A-delta fibres are small diameter, lightly myelinated fibres, which transmit at speeds of between 6 and 30 m/s. They respond to pressure (at any intensity), heat above 45°C (considered the noxious range), chemicals and cooling.
3. C fibres are small diameter, unmyelinated fibres which carry impulses relatively slowly, at speeds of 1–2.5 m/s. In humans they respond to all types of noxious events and as such are considered polymodal (Van Hees and Gybels, 1981; cited in Meyer, Campbell and Raja, 1994). They also respond to light pressure and warmth. They account for 60–70% of all sensory nerve fibres.

Thus noxious stimuli are transmitted via A-delta and C fibres, which will generally require a high intensity stimulus before they are activated. However, it should be remembered that, according to the gate control theory, low intensity stimuli transmitted by A-beta fibres will influence pain perception by blocking the passage of impulses from C and A-delta fibres to the transmission cells in the substantia gelatinosa. Melzack and Wall (1996) suggest that this goes some way toward explaining why a higher frequency of input is required to generate pain from pressure (which would also stimulate A-beta fibres) than from heat (which does not).

If the stimulus is sufficient to trigger an impulse, a series of events associated with the inflammatory response begin a process known as sensitization. Sensitization is characterized by a lowering of the threshold required to generate noxious stimuli, a state known as hyperalgesia. Mediators of the inflammatory response, including prostaglandins and leukotrienes, 5-hydroxytryptamine and histamine, have all been shown to lower the threshold for nociceptor activity (Levine and Taiwo, 1994). The influence of inflammatory mediators helps to account for the more prolonged pain associated with deep tissue injuries such as sprains; pain which continues long after the initial injurious impulse has disappeared and which is stimulated when the injured limb is moved within a range of movement which would not normally cause pain. These findings also help to explain how aspirin and other non-steroidal anti-inflammatory drugs (NSAIDs) exert their analgesic effects. NSAIDs inhibit the production of prostaglandins, substances which both cause pain and stimulate the production of other inflammatory substances which also have a hyperalgesic (pain-enhancing) effect.

It would now seem that even in the absence of actual tissue damage, the transmission of noxious impulses along C fibres may be sufficient to induce an inflammatory response. This effect is mediated by neuropeptides such as substance P which is stored in the neurone cell bodies in the dorsal root ganglion. Stimulation of C fibres results in the release of these peptides peripherally by what has been termed the 'axon reflex' (i.e. the peptides travel down the afferent nerve axon to the source of stimulation). Although substance P does not directly contribute to pain, it does set in motion a series of events which attract other inflammatory agents to the area; substances which either stimulate nerve endings directly or cause sensitization (Rang and Bevan, 1994).

ACTIVITIES IN THE SPINAL CORD

Nerve impulses are delivered via the peripheral C and A-delta fibres to the dorsal horn of the spinal cord. From here they are transferred to ascending sensory fibres for transmission to the brain and other parts of the spinal cord via interneurones. Dorsal horn cells are divided into six laminae (layers) which extend upwards throughout the entire length of the spinal column. The first two laminae are made up of densely packed nerve cells which comprise the substantia gelatinosa. Most of the A-delta and C fibre axons terminate here (Perl, 1980; cited in Melzack and Wall, 1996) and Melzack and Wall proposed it as the site for the gating mechanism responsible for the modification of sensory inputs prior to their transfer to the brain.

The dorsolateral tract descending from the brain innervates most of the dorsal laminae. The tract carries fibres from the raphe nuclei, locus coeruleus, reticular formation and hypothalamus. Other descending tracts may also have fibres which infiltrate the laminae, and in doing so, influence the transfer of noxious stimuli from peripheral fibres to ascending spinal fibres. This is the anatomical basis for the descending inhibitory mechanisms implied in the gate control theory.

The inhibitory processes described above are triggered as soon as pain impulses reach the substantia gelatinosa. Wall (1996) discusses an inhibitory loop which takes more time to generate. This mechanism involves the initiation of impulses within the dorsal horn which ascend to the reticular formation and midbrain. From here the impulses return to the spinal cord via descending tracts. It has been hypothesized that this is a means by which descending control systems are themselves moderated (Schable et al., 1991; cited in Woolf, 1994). It seems logical to presume that the short-fibred interneurones of the dorsal horn transfer pain impulses directly to the brain (excitatory interneurones) or moderate pain impulse transmission (inhibitory interneurones).

Transmission across synapses also requires consideration as inhibitory and excitatory mechanisms may exert their effect by influencing the release and uptake of neurotransmitter substances. A considerable range of substances are released from afferent nerve fibres in response to noxious stimuli. Many of them have the capacity to function as neurotransmitters, but few have been thoroughly investigated (Dickenson, 1996). Interest has tended to focus on the activities of substance P, calcitonin gene-related peptide (CGRP) and excitatory amino acids (glutamate and aspartate).

The role of substance P in promoting peripheral inflammatory events has already been discussed. Substance P is found in C fibres and in interneurones under the influence of descending pathways. Peripheral inflammation is followed by an increase in the release of substance P and another tachykinin peptide: neurokinin A (Duggan et al., 1988; cited in Dickenson, 1996). It is suggested that this induces a central state of hypersensitivity, increasing excitation of fibres within the spinal cord.

CGRP and other peptides have been shown to be released on stimulation of nociceptive afferents and to have an excitatory response on neurones in the dorsal horn. The precise action of CGRP is not know. However, CGRP and substance P are both broken down by the same enzyme. The presence of CGRP in the dorsal horn will leave less of the enzyme available for the breakdown of substance P, thus prolonging the action of substance P.

NEUROTRANSMITTERS

The amino acids glutamate and aspartate are highly influential in the transmission of acute and chronic pain (Dickenson, 1996). Glutamate is a major excitatory neurotransmitter for neurones in the central nervous system. The precise action of glutamate will depend on the receptor activated (a number have been identified). The N-methyl-D-aspartate (NMDA) receptor has provoked considerable interest. Its activation triggers the release of calcium ions into the neurone, substantially increasing excitability to the extent that the activity at this receptor site overrides that at other glutamate receptors. Normally, the NMDA receptor is blocked by magnesium ions which can only be removed by a barrage of afferent impulses. However, the release of peptides which accompanies prolonged or high intensity C fibre activity, facilitates the removal of magnesium ions. This has been widely advocated as a major cause of central hyperalgesia, which may ultimately help to account for some of the chronic pain syndromes (Dickenson, 1996; Melzack and Wall, 1996).

ENDOGENOUS OPIOIDS

Transmission of nerve impulses from sensory afferent fibres to the spinal cord appears also to be under the influence of the body's own morphines (endorphins and enkephalins). Opioid receptors are found both at the periphery and spinal terminals of C fibres and in parts of the brain. When activated, these receptors reduce neuroelectrical activity and limit the release of neurotransmitters, thus reducing the intensity and frequency of impulses reaching ascending spinal tracts. The receptors will respond both to endogenous and pharmacological morphines, but the understanding of the mechanisms by which endorphins are released and receptors activated remains vague.

THE BRAIN'S RESPONSE TO PAIN

Cells in a wide range of brain structures have been found to respond to noxious stimuli (Guilbaud, Bernard and Besson, 1994). This is hardly surprising when one considers that the brain must not only recognize the presence or absence of pain, quantify, qualify and locate it, but must also initiate autonomic and complex learned and afferent (mood associated) responses. The areas most consistently found to change their activity in response to pain include areas of the pons and medulla (especially the dorsal column nuclei, cerebellum and reticular formation), the midbrain (e.g. periaqueductal grey and parabrachial nuclei) and the forebrain (e.g. thalamus, hypothalamus and diverse areas of the cortex). Wall (1996) argues that the search for a few brain centres which might each account for one component of pain (sensory-discriminative, motivational, cognitive/evaluative) is becoming increasingly less practical.

A progression of research projects appears to be providing both the anatomical and physiological basis which lends credence to the gate control theory and which would locate the gating mechanism within the substantia gelatinosa. A summary of the processes involved in pain perception is illustrated in Figure 7.2.

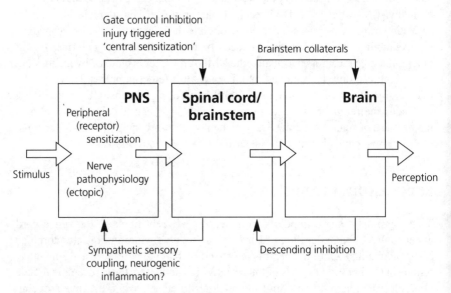

Figure 7.2 Block diagram indicating the major components of the pain system and modulatory relations between them. (From Devor, 1996, p. 104.)

The focus of this chapter has been on the events associated with acute pain experiences. The gate control theory may not on its own account for chronic pain syndromes such as phantom limb pain. However, increasing awareness of the true complexities of acute pain perception makes the dismissal of chronic pain states as psychological phenomena more difficult. It is hoped that this chapter, intended to update the reader on the current thinking in the 'science' of pain, will improve the prospect of treatment for pain sufferers.

References

Devor, M. (1996) Pain mechanisms and pain syndromes, in *Pain 1996; an Updated Review. Refresher Course Syllabus*, (ed. J. N. Campbell), International Association for the Study of Pain, Seattle.

Dickenson A. H. (1996) Pharmacology of pain transmission and control, in *Pain 1996; an Updated Review. Refresher Course Syllabus*, (ed. J. N. Campbell), International Association for the Study of Pain, Seattle.

Guilbaud, G., Bernard J. F. and Besson J. M. (1994) Brain areas involved in nociception and pain, in *Textbook of Pain*, 3rd edn, (eds P. D. Wall and R. Melzack), Churchill Livingstone, Edinburgh.

Levine, J. and Taiwo, Y. (1994) Inflammatory pain, in *Textbook of Pain*, 3rd edn, (eds P. D. Wall and R. Melzack), Churchill Livingstone, Edinburgh.

Melzack, R. and Wall, P. D. (1996) *The Challenge of Pain*, Penguin, London.

Meyer, R. A., Campbell, J. N and Raja, S. N. (1994) Peripheral neural mechanisms of nociception in *Textbook of Pain*, 3rd edn, (eds P. D. Wall and R. Melzack), Churchill Livingstone, Edinburgh.

Rang, H. P. and Bevan, D. A. (1994) Nociceptive peripheral neurons: Cellular properties, in *Textbook of Pain*, 3rd edn, (eds P. D. Wall and R. Melzack), Churchill Livingstone, Edinburgh.

Wall, P. D. (1996) The mechanisms by which tissue damage and pain are related, in *Pain 1996; an Updated Review. Refresher Course Syllabus*, (ed. J. N. Campbell), International Association for the Study of Pain, Seattle.

Woolf, C. J. (1994) The dorsal horn: state-dependent sensory processing and the generation of pain, in *Textbook of Pain*, 3rd edn, (eds P. D. Wall and R. Melzack), Churchill Livingstone, Edinburgh.

<table>
<tr><td>**8**</td><td># Pain therapies</td></tr>
</table>

Excellent herbs had our fathers of old –
Excellent herbs to ease their pain.

Our Fathers of Old
Kipling

… happily the effects of two or more therapies given in combination are cumulative.

Melzack and Wall, 1996

In this chapter the reader is introduced to some of the most widely used therapies in the management of pain. This topic forms the largest chapter in the book but in fact only touches the tip of the iceberg and really represents only an overview of the subject. By the time the book is in print no doubt new therapies, new devices and new analgesics will have appeared on the market. The reader is encouraged to try and keep abreast of current trends in pain treatments.

So far, this book has focused on the complex nature of pain. The traditional approach to treating pain has been to use invasive methods; that is to say, methods that physically invade or enter the body. Examples of these are analgesic drugs, nerve blocks or surgical procedures. Increasingly, however, it is being recognized that, because so many factors influence the nature of pain, both the local tissue damage and innumerable external factors, it is best to treat pain (acute or chronic) using a combined physical and psychological approach. This approach (known as the biopsychosocial approach) is not only wise but imperative in the management of chronic pain. It is also recognized that while acute pain can be completely controlled, pain of a chronic nature is less easily managed. So that while both types of pain may be managed using the same or similar treatments, chronic pain responds less well and on the whole is less well understood by health professionals.

Most of the therapies outlined below could easily be used in an integrated way. Some of them lie directly within the province of most health professionals; for example, distraction techniques, guided imagery and relaxation are all non-invasive methods that nurses can initiate without a doctor's prescription. If a particular method does not work it can be discarded. It should be accepted by health professionals that pain in different people responds differently to different treatments. The patient should not be 'blamed' if a particular treatment does not work. The nurse should try to individualize each approach to suit a particular patient and his pain. Sometimes patients can be taught to use certain techniques without help.

Nurses do not generally prescribe medications, although this is changing in relation to prescribing of mild analgesics and some other medications in community settings. Nurses do, though, have considerable 'power' in relation to the administration of analgesics. In this respect, nurses must be familiar with the rules regarding administration and the possible side effects of drugs. Nurses also do not carry out local anaesthetic blocks, but they do have a role in preparing and supporting patients throughout this and other invasive treatments.

DISTRACTION

Distraction is when someone focuses attention on a stimulus other than the pain. Sometimes distraction can or has to be used without planning or explanation. On other occasions, a nurse may plan beforehand and rehearse with a patient a particularly useful strategy prior to a painful procedure. It may be helpful to boost the confidence of a patient by taking an opportunity to practise while he is pain free. The quality of the nurse–patient relationship will influence the patient's willingness to try a particular technique.

Some patients use distraction themselves, without being taught, but do not tell the staff that they are consciously doing so. Reading, listening to music or watching television are examples of distraction. Imagination (mental imagery) is another form of distraction. Distraction may increase a patient's tolerance for pain and sometimes decrease the intensity of pain. What seems to happen is that pain ceases to be the focus of the patient's attention.

Unfortunately, as Weiner (1975) noted over 20 years ago, many health professionals doubt that a patient is in pain if he is able to distract himself or be distracted. This still sometimes seems to be the case. One comment recently overheard from a nurse was that a patient was 'sitting up in bed chatting happily to visitors', the assumption being that the patient could not possibly have been experiencing much pain. Perhaps the patient was being distracted from his pain. In one early study it was found that patients developed their own coping behaviours at home but felt that doctors or nurses 'might not like it'. They felt that their coping behaviours might be 'against the rules' and might be laughed at as not being scientific (Copp, 1974). Payne and Walker (1996) noted that past experiences of coping with stressful situations shape future responses. This was obvious with one patient who was interviewed by Sofaer (1984). She was an elderly Scottish lady who had 'been through two world wars'. She declined any analgesia offered to her following surgery on both feet. When asked how she managed, she replied, 'I knew what I had to do to distract myself from the pain'.

Following the use of distraction, increased awareness of pain and fatigue may be present. A patient should therefore be offered an appropriate alternative method of relief following distraction. Another approach is to use distraction consciously while waiting for other methods to take effect. One patient said, 'I listen to music while waiting for the painkillers to take effect'.

Distraction alone is a potent pain reliever in certain situations. For example, when changing dressings, nurses can distract patients by getting them to talk about a favourite pastime, a book they may be reading, or their family. If patients do not feel like talking when in pain, another useful strategy is for the nurse to suggest to the patient that he stares at a spot (anything close at hand, from a flower to a door knob) during which an area of skin is massaged in a slow, rhythmic, often circular manner. The nurse can do this or the patient can do it for himself. The massage can be done on or near the painful area or on another part of the body, depending on the nature of the injury. Another distraction strategy involves slow, rhythmic breathing.

A method of distraction frequently used with children is to read stories to them and get them to describe the pictures. Adult patients can also do this, by looking at pictures of particular interest, and using their senses in an imaginative way. For example, while looking at a picture of a country scene, the patient could imagine he hears the birds singing, feels the warmth of the sun on his skin and smells the fragrant flowers. This is using imagery in conjunction with distraction.

IMAGERY

The technique of imagery is different insofar as distraction is usually dependent on external stimuli, whereas imagery depends on the mind exclusively, usually through evoking visual sensations, although best results may be obtained by using all the senses. Imagery may be taught to a patient for distraction purposes. It may be preceded by a relaxation technique (p. 89). Imagery, as taught to a patient for self-use, gives the patient control over whether he will use it and when. In using imagery, the patient is alert and concentrating very hard.

One example of the power of imagery is to imagine yourself slicing a lemon and arranging it on a dish. When did your mouth begin to water? Imagination seems to involve responses from both mind and body.

Progressive relaxation exercises, followed by imagining idyllic scenes, may be useful in relieving both acute and chronic pain. A colleague with a severe migraine tried the following technique until he was able to get to a pharmacy and purchase medication. He imagined himself near a beach – he did not like the sun so he chose the shade of a tree under which to rest. When asked what he heard, smelled and felt, he replied that he had 'heard the sound of the waves and of children playing, smelled the sea air and felt the breeze on my face'. This imagery took about 15 minutes, by which time he had reached a pharmacy. It is useful to find out from a patient to what extent he already uses imagery as a pain-relieving technique and it should be pointed out that imagery can be used along with other pain-relieving techniques.

If you guide the imagery you can use persuasive suggestions. For instance, you could say, 'When you are ready' or 'Perhaps you feel' (for example, the warmth of the sun). This approach involves the patient in deciding what is best for him. Sometimes people feel drowsy afterwards. If the patient wants to sleep he can say to himself, 'When I awake I will feel fresh'. If he does not want to sleep, he could suggest to himself that when he has finished his imagining he will feel alert and awake.

Imagery can be used either for very brief periods or for a longer time, perhaps up to 20 minutes. One way to encourage a patient to use imagery is for the nurse to suggest to the patient that he pictures himself in a pleasant environment, for example in a park. The nurse can then ask the patient for a description of his surroundings, encouraging responses that use all his senses. If the patient has difficulty, the nurse could help by introducing appropriate images. For example, for one patient who was feeling very hot, it was suggested that she imagine herself resting under the shade of a big, leafy tree, feeling the cool breeze. Visual imagery can also be very helpful during uncomfortable procedures such as removal of sutures.

One specific image for pain relief involves picturing the pain flowing away from the body. This was described by McCaffery (1983, p. 262) as the instructions she gives to a patient with a tension headache. For patients with pain in another site, the word 'head' can be replaced with the appropriate site. The book is now out of print but it is still available in many nursing libraries. The instructions are as follows.

Get into a comfortable position. Close your eyes. Now, take a slow, rather deep breath and feel yourself relax as you breathe out. Continue to breathe comfortably and slowly, feeling your body relax each time you breathe out. If you wish, the next time you breathe in you can imagine that your breath goes to your head, bringing nutrients, comfort and calm. As you breathe out, you can imagine that the air goes out through your head, taking with it the discomfort, leaving behind relaxed, healthy, comfortable tissues. Each time you breathe in you can picture the air flowing through to your head, bringing health and comfort. As you breathe out, the air once again flows out through your head, leaving calm, relaxation, health and comfort behind. I will pause now and you can continue to breathe slowly and imagine more and more comfort with each breath that flows through your head (pause for whatever amount of time seems reasonable, for example, 15, five or one minute). When you are ready, you may end this image by counting silently to yourself from one to three. At the count of three inhale, open your eyes and say to yourself that you feel alert and relaxed. I will wait now until you are ready to end this for yourself. Take your time. Enjoy the experience.

One variation is for the patient to imagine he is sitting on a river bank and with each breath out his pain flows down the river and out to sea.

Another image that may be useful is for the patient to imagine himself as healthy. The nurse can suggest to the patient the following short image as also described by McCaffery (1983).

If you wish, you may begin to picture yourself as being healthy. Perhaps you would like to begin with your toes and slowly work upwards. You may find this easier to do with your eyes closed. You may see each part of your body form- ing just as you want it to be. You can paint this picture of yourself in your mind's eye or you can simply allow the picture to form slowly. You can see that each body part is healthy. See yourself exactly as you want to be. See yourself healed. See each part of yourself functioning normally, inside and outside your body.

Using imagery with children can be particularly helpful. It could be the 'let's pre- tend' game. Allowing the child to imagine being his favourite hero in a story may be an acceptable way of helping a child to cope with pain. For an excellent source on managing pain in children, the reader is referred to Carter (1994).

The use of colour, either in the environment or imagination, may be helpful to both children and adults. One patient used six coloured bangles as an aid to help her imagine the sun, sea and earth and was able to create some very beautiful images for herself.

RELAXATION TECHNIQUES

Relaxation exercises used in conjunction with imagery may enhance the effect of the imagery.

Relaxation is freedom from mental and physical tension and stress. There are several techniques available to achieve a state of relaxation, all requiring the patient's participation. One or more techniques may often be combined with other therapies such as counselling to make a programme that may sometimes be referred to as relaxation therapy. Described below are individual techniques, any of which may also be used prior to using imagery to enhance its effect.

Many patients already practise some form of relaxation technique. The nurse should enquire about this and if a patient finds a particular technique helpful, the nurse should encourage its use.

Relaxation may be achieved by various means – for example, meditation, yoga or progressive relaxation exercises. Whatever technique is used, the aim should be to reduce the effect of stress. It is not clear how stress and pain are related but it may be that stress aggravates pain. It is, however, generally recognized that there is a relationship between pain, tension and anxiety. Relaxation techniques may also help to lower anxiety. This may, in certain circumstances, be helpful to over-anxious patients. A further point is that a relaxation technique can act as a distraction so that the patient's mind is taken off the pain. Muscle relaxation training has been found to decrease 'state anxiety', that is anxiety which may be present in patients facing potentially stressful events (Johnson and Spielberger, 1968). Relaxation may help a patient to sleep. Since pain is fatiguing it is a useful strategy in overcoming fatigue.

Some people have erroneous beliefs that relaxing is achieved by reading a book or watching television. In these situations, a person may still feel stressed. It is important to realize that people need to learn relaxation techniques. It is helpful if one can choose a quiet environment and assume a comfortable position to practise relaxation. Some people like to lie down, others prefer to sit in a straight-backed chair.

A technique recommended by McCaffery (1983), which can be accomplished quickly, is to:

1. breathe in deeply and clench your fists;
2. breathe out and go limp as a rag doll;
3. start yawning.

Repeat these instructions as often as necessary. Step 1 should always be followed by Step 2, but Steps 2 and 3 can be repeated alone at intervals.

Slow, rhythmic breathing can also be effective. It is often helpful for patients who experience chronic pain and who may like to use some method of relaxation regularly. The nurse can teach the patient to do abdominal breathing and then instruct them as follows.

1. Close your eyes and take a slow, deep breath.
2. As you breathe out, feel yourself relax. Feel the tension draining out of your body.
3. Breathe slowly and comfortably from your abdomen.
4. Think about your breathing. Feel the air enter your nose and lungs. Feel the air go out of your lungs and feel yourself relaxing as you breathe out.
5. To help you breathe slowly and rhythmically, as you inhale I will say 'in, one, two'; as you exhale, 'out, one, two'. (Say these phrases in co-ordination with the patient's breathing in and out. Do this two or three times to help the patient slow his breathing and keep it regular.)
6. Feel yourself relax each time you breathe out. Just let the air flow from your lungs and let the tension flow from your body.
7. As you breathe in you may say silently to yourself, 'in, one, two'. As you

breathe out you may say to yourself, 'relax'. (Say these phrases two or three times in co-ordination with the patient's breathing. A word other than 'relax' may have been chosen by the patient prior to using the technique.)

8. I am going to pause now to let you concentrate on your breathing. Relax as you breathe out, breathing slowly and rhythmically, counting silently for yourself if you wish. (Watch the patient and if tension or difficulty arises, begin the counting for him and repeat the instructions in step 7.)

9. When you are ready to end this relaxation you may do so yourself. When you are ready, count silently from one to three. At the count of three, inhale deeply, silently say to yourself, 'I feel alert and relaxed', and open your eyes. I will wait now for you to end your relaxation for yourself when you are ready.

It may be helpful for some patients if the nurse puts the instructions on tape, possibly including some guided imagery. For home-care patients this may be particularly useful since they could play the tape whenever they felt the need. An earpiece may be used so as not to disturb other patients or, if at home, members of a family.

Some problems may occasionally arise. For example, a person may become very aware of body sensations or become withdrawn. Alternatively, patients may complain that techniques are 'boring'. Perhaps modifying the technique would help. If not, the nurse should discuss with the patient the possibility of discontinuing its use.

ANALGESICS

The administration of analgesic drugs is a common method of pain relief. Because doctors prescribe the drugs, it is sometimes assumed that understanding them is solely a medical responsibility. However, it is particularly important that nurses, too, understand how analgesics work since it is to nurses that patients will most often turn for pain relief. Control of pain often depends on nursing staff, for nurses hold the keys of the cupboard where analgesics are kept. Nurses can exercise their discretion so that patients have the maximum control of pain. Too often, the power that nurses have in this respect is used negatively, without individual assessment of pain and without any knowledge of drug potency. One example to illustrate this idea is that frequently nurses administer drugs at drug round times in a ritualistic way, not talking to patients in between drug rounds about their pain or assessing pain levels. Nurses must also take responsibility for consulting medical colleagues whenever they are in doubt or whenever they need help in managing pain. This should go without saying, but is being said because unless there is co-operation and communication, patients will inevitably suffer pain unnecessarily.

However, there are increasing examples of good practice and many hospitals now have protocols for relief of pain following surgery. An example of how one hospital has introduced protocols for optimizing analgesia postoperatively is summarized on p. 101. The reader is urged to read it and note that medication is not restricted to 'four-hourly'. 'Four-hourly' is an unfortunate term that has crept into prescribing, but in the case of postoperative pain control particularly, there is huge variation in experience of efficacy of drugs between different people.

In discussing potency, a distinction is drawn between opioid analgesics and non-opioid analgesics. Opioid analgesics work by acting on the central nervous system, whereas non-opioid analgesics act on the nerves at the site of pain. Opiates such as morphine are usually the only drugs effective in combating severe pain, whereas non-opioid analgesics such as aspirin are helpful for relief of mild to moderate pain. Some types of pain, such as bone pain, are not responsive to opiates.

The ideal analgesic drug should be easily administered, effective, safe and inexpensive. The most important criterion is safety but, as with all drugs, the use of both opioids and non-opioids carries risks. Some commonly used opioid and non-opioid analgesic drugs are described below, but this is by no means a comprehensive list and is only intended as an introduction to the subject. Latham (1990) has written an excellent chapter on the use of drugs in pain control. Nurses particularly are encouraged to read it.

Opiates

Opioid analgesics affect perception of pain by acting on the central nervous system. They are used to relieve severe pain and also may produce a sense of well-being. Opioids include both natural and synthetic drugs and are also known as opiates or morphine and its congeners. They act on morphine receptors. Opioid analgesics are subject to the provisions of the Misuse of Drugs Act 1971 and have to be prescribed by a medical or dental practitioner. They are therefore called controlled drugs.

The 1985 Misuse of Drugs Regulations has specified the classes of people who are authorized to supply and possess controlled drugs in their capacity as professionals. Drugs are controlled depending on their formulation. Five schedules are identified in the regulations. Schedules two and three particularly apply to analgesics. Schedule two drugs are those which are subject to full control. They have to be prescribed in writing, kept in safe custody and recorded in registers. Examples include morphine, diamorphine and pethidine. Schedule three drugs require a special prescription but are not subject to safe custody or register requirements. A requirement is that invoices have to be kept for two years. Drugs which come under these regulations include buprenorphine and also oral pentazocine, which is rarely prescribed.

There are two types of regulation regarding administration of drugs: first, Statutory Regulations relating to Acts of Parliament, and, second, local hospital regulations. Individual health authorities also draw up guidelines for storage and administration of medicines. Doses referred to below are adult doses given in the *British National Formulary* (1997).

Morphine

The most commonly used opiate is morphine, a derivative of opium. The duration of action of morphine is usually considered to be about four hours, but this should not be taken for granted because of individual variation. The usual dose for an adult is 10 mg administered intramuscularly or subcutaneously 1–4-hourly. Pain relief following administration should be assessed according to the guidelines in Chapter 5. Please also consult the example of a protocol for relief of postoperative pain on p. 101. Different routes of administration will result in different potencies. Intramuscular, intravenous and subcutaneous administration for acute pain control are thought to be six times more potent than the oral route and in chronic pain control, three times more potent (Latham, 1990). Morphine may also be administered via the epidural route where it is thought to be ten times more potent than the oral route and intrathecally where it is 100 times more potent than the oral route.

The major side effect of morphine is dose-related respiratory depression. Care is needed in situations where this could be dangerous, e.g. in patients with pulmonary disease. Overdose of morphine can suppress respiration completely and cause death. The depressant effect of morphine on the respiratory system can be counteracted by administering a specific morphine antagonist. The drug of choice for reversing this effect is naloxone.

Other side effects of morphine may be nausea and/or vomiting with the initial doses. Usually, therefore, an antiemetic drug is prescribed with morphine. Oral morphine is suitable for relief of pain in terminal care. A simple elixir of morphine and water may be prescribed together with an antiemetic such as prochlorperazine. A dose of 20–30 mg of morphine in an oral solution is generally considered to be equivalent to 10 mg of morphine by injection. Morphine can also be administered by rectum using suppositories. These come in 10–30 mg strengths. A sustained-release form of morphine is available in tablet form (MST Continus, 5–200 mg strengths). This is a long-acting preparation which may be helpful in the relief of prolonged and severe pain. The dose is dependent on the severity of the pain.

Morphine induces constriction of the pupils of the eyes. It also decreases peristaltic activity of the gastrointestinal tract. One side-effect of this is constipation, which is inevitable with the use of opioids, and patients need strong stimulant laxatives. If someone is going to be given opioids for more than 24 hours, they should be given laxatives routinely. Further possible side effects are lowering of blood pressure, dizziness and itching of the skin. One feature of morphine therapy is the development of patient tolerance; that is, the need to administer increasingly large doses to produce the same analgesic effect. If clinical tolerance develops, it is important to realize that this cannot be equated with addiction. There is also no reason to believe that it will lead to addiction (Jaffe, 1975). Drug abuse is a voluntary behaviour. Drug tolerance and physical dependence are involuntary behaviours based on physiological changes that take place within the body.

Diamorphine (Heroin)

Diamorphine is a derivative of morphine. Following administration, diamorphine has a more rapid onset and shorter duration than that of morphine. It causes less nausea and hypotension. The usual dose is 5–10 mg given intramuscularly or subcutaneously. Diamorphine can also be given in oral solution, 13–20 mg given orally being equivalent to 4–5 mg by injection. Diamorphine can cause greater respiratory depression than morphine. It can be administered epidurally, intrathecally and intravenously. It is more effective than morphine because it is more lipid soluble.

Papaveretum (Omnopon)

Papaveretum is given to relieve moderate to severe pain. It does not appear to have any advantage over morphine. It consists of 253 parts of morphine hydrochloride, 23 parts of papaverine hydrochloride and 20 parts of codeine hydrochloride. It can be given by injection, subcutaneously, intramuscularly or intravenously. It is prescribed as 7.7 mg/ml or 15.4 mg/ml; the higher dose provides the equivalent of 10mg of morphine. It has muscle relaxant properties and is often used as a premedication and as an analgesic postoperatively.

Pethidine

This is a synthetic opioid drug unrelated to morphine. It is a powerful analgesic that also reduces muscle spasm. It is very useful for the treatment of renal and biliary colic and labour pain. The usual dose is 50–100 mg given intramuscularly. Following administration, the onset of its effect is rapid, but duration of action is shorter than morphine, usually about 2–3 hours. There may be less respiratory depression than with morphine, but pethidine should not be given to patients who are taking psychotropic drugs of the monoamine oxidase inhibitor group as excitation, coma, changes in blood pressure or death could occur. As with morphine, tolerance and dependence can develop. It is available in both injection and tablet form and also parenterally (without preservatives) for use as epidural or intrathethcal administration. The oral dose is 50–150 mg.

Dihydrocodeine tartrate (DF118)

Dihydrocodeine tartrate (DF118) is administered orally (30–60 mg) or intramuscularly (50 mg). If given intramuscularly, it is regarded as a controlled drug; if given orally, it is not. It is used for the relief of moderate to severe pain. Side effects are dizziness, nausea and constipation.

Codeine phosphate

Codeine phosphate is administered orally (15–30 mg) or intramuscularly (up to 30 mg). Tolerance and dependence are common. Side effects are dizziness, nausea, and constipation. It is useful for treating head injuries as it is said not to cause progressive sedation with increasing doses.

Phenazocine (Narphen)

This analgesic is effective for severe pain, particularly biliary colic and pancreatic pain. It is less likely to increase biliary pressure than other analgesics. Nausea and vomiting may occur and if so the drug can be administered sublingually. The oral dose is 5 mg four-hourly but a single dose may be given as 20 mg.

Methadone (Physeptone)

Methadone may be administered for severe pain. It is less effective and sedating than morphine. It is sometimes used for the relief of terminal pain. The injections may cause local pain and tissue damage. The usual dose is 5–10 mg which can be administered subcutaneously or intramuscularly. By mouth the dose is usually 20 mg. Methadone may have a greater respiratory depressant effect than morphine. In some situations it is used to suppress intractable cough and dyspnoea and can be used to treat a cough in terminal illness. One problem with methadone is that it has an accumulative effect if given over a long time. The patient's tolerance does not increase as it does with morphine.

Buprenorphine (Temgesic)

Buprenorphine is used to treat moderate to severe pain. The side effects are less marked than those of morphine, although it may be helpful to give an antiemetic over the first few days of administration. The effects of buprenorphine may not be reversed by naloxone. It may therefore antagonize analgesia from large doses of morphine and should not be given to patients who have become tolerant to morphine since withdrawal symptoms could result. Buprenorphine is administered sublingually in 200 µg tablets or by intramuscular injection (300 µg).

Dextromoramide (Palfium)

This is a very short-acting opioid (2–3 hours' duration). It is useful as an extra for occasional breakthrough pain or before a painful procedure.

Pentazocine (Fortral)

Pentazocine, a partial opioid agonist/antagonist, is used to relieve moderate to severe pain. It is administered orally, 25–100 mg after food, or by subcutaneous, intramuscular or intravenous injection, 30–60 mg. Rectal suppositories (50 mg) are also available. Side effects include mild respiratory depression, nausea, vomiting, dizziness and hallucinations.

Compound preparations

There are several combination drugs which are frequently used for moderate pain. Doses are usually 1–2 tablets 4–6-hourly.

Dextropropoxyphene hydrochloride and paracetamol (Co-proxamol)

Each tablet consists of dextropropoxyphene 32.5 mg and paracetamol 325 mg.

Dihydrocodeine tartrate and paracetamol (Co-dydramol)

Each tablet consists of dihydrocodeine tartrate 10 mg and paracetamol 500 mg.

Codeine phosphate and aspirin (Co-codaprin)

Each tablet or dispersible tablet consists of codeine phosphate 8 mg and aspirin 400 mg.

Codeine phosphate and paracetamol

Each tablet or dispersible tablet consists of codeine phosphate 8 mg and paracetamol 500 mg.

Aspirin and papaveretum (Aspav)

Each dispersible tablet consists of papaveretum 5 mg and aspirin 500 mg. It can be used very successfully to control postoperative pain three or four days following major surgery but may need to be taken in conjunction with a drug to prevent gastric irritation, such as ranitidine or omeprazole.

Intravenous opioids

In Great Britain, nurses do not usually give intravenous injections of opioids. However, in some units, they may do so when there is an agreement with medical staff. Intravenous injections of opioids are given slowly, over a 3–5-minute period, and the effect is almost immediate. The duration of action is, however, shorter than when an opioid is given intramuscularly.

Infusion pumps

Analgesics may be administered by means of an infusion pump. There are a number of infusion pumps available for use in different situations. Routes of administration also may vary depending on the situation. Intravenous analgesic infusions may be used in the management of postoperative pain, whereas subcutaneous infusion is more often used in palliative care. In some hospitals, subcutaneous infusions of opioids are used for postoperative analgesia. With the latter, the cannula may be placed in the chest, upper arm or abdomen.

Local policy for administration of analgesics using infusion pumps varies between hospitals. One example of a local policy for optimizing postoperative analgesia appears at the end of the section on management of acute pain using analgesic drugs (p. 101).

For more information on infusion sets, care of the skin and how to use portable infusion pumps, the reader is referred to Latham (1990).

Sandler (1994) noted that now there are so many postoperative analgesic techniques, the best choice for each patient is not always clear. Two of the most commonly used methods, epidural infusions and patient-controlled analgesic systems, sometimes called patient-controlled administration (PCA), are described below. Sandler also pointed out that there may be a relationship between specific psychological factors and satisfaction with PCA; for example, Vickers (1985) noted patient satisfaction with PCA was predicted by locus of control beliefs. Patients who scored highly on an internal locus of control scale showed lower pain scores and higher levels of satisfaction with PCA. (Locus of control is discussed in Chapter 3.) Effective use of PCA devices requires that patients believe that one's health is in one's own hands. On the other hand, as Egan and Ready (1994) found, a main disadvantage of the use of PCA can be the lack of effective analgesia immediately following surgery and prior to PCA being instituted. They also found that patients who had epidural anaesthesia appreciated having a clear mind and having effective relief at rest and while coughing or mobilizing.

Epidural infusions

Epidural infusions are useful in the management of acute pain, for example labour pain or postoperative pain, and preoperatively prior to amputation in an attempt to reduce postoperative phantom pain. Usually epidural infusions are commenced in the anaesthetic room and used in conjunction with general anaesthesia or alone to manage pain both during and following surgery. The idea behind the epidural infusion is to block sensory nerve pathways and thus prevent pain. Some degree of motor block can affect the ability of the patient to mobilize. This usually wears off. There are a variety of drugs which can be used but the main one is bupivacaine (Marcain). Sometimes combinations of drugs are used, i.e. bupivacaine with diamorphine or with fentanyl or pethidine.

Patients having an epidural infusion should be monitored closely by nursing staff for respiration rate, if an opioid is being administered, and blood pressure volume because of the possible vasodilatory effects of a local anaesthetic on the sympathetic nervous system. In addition, patients need to be monitored for urinary output to ensure that renal insufficiency or retention (due to sensory loss) does not occur. Also, the nurse needs to watch for other side effects including nausea, vomiting and itching, all of which can be easily treated. While assessing for pain relief, it is important that the nurse checks for unwanted lower limb blockade.

Patient-controlled analgesia

Patient-controlled analgesic therapy (PCA) is a method of intravenous opioid administration suitable for adults who are rational and not in circulatory shock. It requires purpose-built equipment in which a previously programmed drug injector is connected to a venous cannula in the patient's arm or hand. A pre-set dose of opioid (e.g. 1–3 mg of morphine) can then be delivered over a predetermined time, when the patient feels the need for it, by the patient himself activating a press-button switch. Once a bolus dose has been administered by the patient, the infusion pump is programmed to go into 'lockout'. During this time (3–15 minutes) no further medication can be obtained by the patient. This is a safety feature. In one study where this method was used postoperatively, patients experienced better pain relief than would have occurred with conventional intramuscular administration and respiratory depression was not found to be a problem (Keeri-Szanto and Heaman, 1972). In addition, it has been reported that patients are enthusiastic about the method and that side effects are minimal (Tamsen et al., 1982).

Different manufacturers provide different options but all machines should have the facility for patients to give their own bolus doses and in special circumstances to be programmed to give a continuous infusion. Nurses must ensure that the patient fully understands and is able to use the PCA. Effective use will soon become apparent if the nurse carries out regular pain assessment. As well as being aware of the possible side effects of the opioid drugs being used, the nurse should also ensure that the patient is assessed for rate and volume of respirations, increasing sedation and any developing nausea, all of which, if detected early, can be treated. A PCA is most effective when it helps the patient to mobilize.

Lynch et al. (1997) noted that in studies where single surgical procedures were carried out, it was found that epidural and PCA were the most satisfactory methods of analgesia. They suggested however, that whatever method is used, pain control needs to be more aggressive, particularly during mobilization.

Counteracting respiratory depressant effects of narcotics

When opioids are in use, an opioid antagonist such as naloxone should always be available in case opioid-induced respiratory depression develops. Naloxone is the drug most commonly used to counteract respiratory depression. Care should be taken not to precipitate withdrawal symptoms and not to counteract all the analgesia afforded by the opioid. The suggested dose is 100–200 µg (1.5–3 µg/kg), adjusted according to the response of the patient, and then 100 µg every two minutes. The nurse must continue to observe a patient following administration of naloxone as the duration of action of this drug may be as short as 30 minutes, whereas the depressant effects of some opioids may be considerably longer. Repeated treatments with naloxone may therefore be required.

Generally speaking, it is safe to give a patient enough opioid to relieve pain but, unfortunately, many patients suffer unrelieved pain due to the inadequate use of opioid analgesics. This may be for a variety of reasons including underprescribing, failure to understand the importance of the individual nature of pain and, in the treatment of acute pain and the pain of terminal illness, a misplaced fear of addiction by health professionals.

Non-opioid analgesics

Non-opioid analgesics such as aspirin and paracetamol are useful in the relief of musculoskeletal pain and most types of moderate to mild pain and as an adjunct prescription for pain from bone secondaries in patients with malignant disease.

Non-steroidal anti-inflammatory drugs (NSAIDs)

Aspirin

Aspirin has an anti-inflammatory action and acts quickly. One difficulty with this analgesic is gastric irritation, but less irritant buffered preparations are available. It should not be given to patients with gastrointestinal problems, with haemophilia or those who are on anticoagulant therapy, since irritation can be sufficient to cause gastric haemorrhage. The dose is 30–900 mg every 4–6 hours when necessary. The maximum daily dose is 4 g.

Diflunisal (Dolobid)

The contraindications for this drug are the same as for aspirin. The dose is 250–500 mg. Tablets should be swallowed whole. Absorption is reduced if the drug is given in conjunction with an antacid.

Mefenamic acid (Ponstan)

This drug is used to treat mild to moderate pain. It should not be given to patients with peptic ulceration or inflammatory conditions of the bowel, those with renal or hepatic impairment or pregnant women. It may cause drowsiness, dizziness, gastric disturbances and diarrhoea. The dose is 500 mg taken orally after food.

Ibuprofen

Ibuprofen is used in the treatment of pain and inflammation in rheumatic disease and other musculoskeletal disorders. The dose is 200–400 mg given orally in tablet form.

Diclofenac sodium (Voltarol)

This is used to treat renal colic and biliary colic and also following major surgery. It is a very effective drug. It can be given IM or by suppository and should not cause drowsiness. The daily dose is 75–150 mg in divided doses by tablet, slow release tablet, injection or rectal suppository. The maximum daily dose is 150 mg.

Other drugs

Paracetamol

This drug is similar in effect to aspirin but it has no anti-inflammatory action. It is less irritant to the gastrointestinal tract than aspirin. Overdose may cause liver damage which may not be obvious for up to six days. The dose is 0.5–1 g, either in the form of tablets or as an elixir.

Carbamazepine (Tegretol)

Although not strictly an analgesic, this drug is very effective in the treatment of trigeminal neuralgia.

Amitriptyline

This is a tricyclic antidepressant drug and works as an adjuvant in certain nerve pains.

Topical preparations

NSAIDs

There are a variety of topical preparations which are useful for the relief of soft-tissue inflammation. These include preparations such as Feldene gel and Voltarol gel.

Counterirritants

Axsain cream is used in the treatment of postherpetic neuralgia after the lesions have healed. Local anaesthetic applications such as Emla are usually used pre-emptively and prior to a painful procedure being carried out. They are particularly useful for children.

Analgesic laddering

The concept of step laddering should be used in conjunction with assessment for all types of pain.

Severe pain
Morphine
Diamorphine
Pethidine
Tramadol
Aspirin and papaveretum (Aspav)

Moderate pain
Codeine
Tylex or Solpadol (paracetamol+ 30 mg codeine)
Dihydrocodeine
Buprenorphine
Meptazinol
Nefopam
NSAIDs, e.g. Voltarol

Mild pain
Co-codamol
Co-dydramol
Co-proxamol
Co-codaprin
Aspirin
Paracetamol

Figure 8.1 Ladder of analgesic drugs showing increasing analgesic potency.

New analgesics are constantly appearing on the market and it is important that nurses appreciate the action of new drugs and know about possible side effects. Detailed information can be found in pharmacology textbooks. The *British National Formulary* gives up-to-date information and nurses must be familiar with consulting it.

One newly available analgesic is trans-dermal fentanyl. It is used presently in the treatment of cancer pain but also in some instances of severe chronic (non-malignant) pain.

The management of acute pain using analgesic drugs

In treating acute pain, a preventive approach is useful. Analgesics should be given before pain returns to prevent severe pain. Analgesics should, however, be viewed as part of an overall pain control strategy that includes a variety of measures, some of which may be taught to the patient. In individualizing management of acute pain, the nurse should observe a patient's response to a treatment and be prepared to discuss possible adjustments in dose if analgesics are being given.

Intramuscular or intravenous routes may be used for severe pain, changing to oral, sublingual or rectal routes when the intensity of the pain subsides. The choice of route depends on the medication prescribed and on the nature of the injury or operation site. However, nurses should recognize the dangers of changing to less potent analgesics too soon. (Note comments on the protocol below.) When an analgesic is not effective in terms of duration of pain, shortening the interval between administrations will be of help rather than adding a drug to sedate.

Nurses should always be aware of the possibility of undertreating pain and the importance of frequent assessment with the patient.

The fear of addiction is not well founded in the treatment of acute pain with opioids. Undertreatment may in fact increase the likelihood of 'clock watching' – that is, when a patient waits expectantly for the next dose of analgesia. This kind of situation can lead to psychological problems. The answer to avoiding this lies in providing adequate pain control.

Accident and emergency treatment

The majority of patients who attend A&E do so because of injury or illness (Selbst and Clarke, 1990). It is important that staff assess and treat the pain as well as assessing and treating the injury/illness.

Particularly in A&E, Entonox (a 50/50 mixture of nitrous oxide and oxygen from one cylinder) may be used advantageously. It is rapidly effective and can be self-administered.

Grant (1997) found that although nurses in A&E departments held an awareness about pain management, they felt that on the whole pain was not well managed due to lack of time, staff and knowledge.

Optimizing postoperative analgesia. Synopses of protocols from the Conquest Hospital, Hastings, East Sussex (reproduced with permission)

- *Intramuscular:* morphine is the first choice where age is under 65 years. The dose is 10 mg hourly PRN. Pethidine (used when morphine is unsuitable, particularly in the elderly) 75–100 mg hourly PRN.
- *PCA:* once again, the first choice of drug is morphine with a bolus dose of 1 mg and lockout of five minutes. The second choice, should morphine be contraindicated, is pethidine, with a bolus dose of 10 mg and a lockout of five minutes.
- *Epidural:* bupivacaine (Marcain) 0.15% with 10 mg diamorphine running at a rate of 3–10 ml per hour. As a second choice, fentanyl 500 µg can be used in place of diamorphine.

Whatever the route of administration, it is important that pain is assessed at regular intervals and doses adjusted accordingly.

The concept of 'balanced analgesia' is useful in controlling postoperative pain. Using more than one class of drug can be helpful to maximize analgesia and minimize side effects. Sometimes it is helpful to give an opioid along with a non-opioid analgesic. For example, one can add a compound analgesic and/or NSAIDs (rectally or orally) to opioid IM or PCA or epidural analgesia.

The management of chronic pain using analgesics and other drugs

The management of chronic pain presents an entirely different problem. Patients suffering chronic pain fall into two groups. First, those suffering persistent pain with a normal expectation of life and, second, those who have a short expectation of life and are suffering from malignant disease. In the latter case, pain is continuous and becomes worse. Because of the short life expectancy, the possibility of addiction to opioids is not important. These patients should be given analgesia in sufficient strength, quantity, and frequency to control their pain (Lipton, 1979; Twycross, 1994).

It is increasingly common practice in palliative medicine to use the guidelines of the WHO for the relief of cancer pain. If, after assessment of the patient, drug therapy is decided upon, four categories of basic drugs are used:

1. non-opioids such as aspirin or paracetamol or non-steroidal anti-inflammatory drugs such as ibuprofen;
2. weak opioids such as codeine or dextropropoxyphene;
3. strong opioids such as morphine, pethidine or buprenorphine;
4. adjuvants, which include anticonvulsants, such as carbamazepine; neuroleptics, such as prochlorperazine and haloperidol; anxiolytics, such as diazepam; antidepressants, such as amitriptyline; corticosteroids, such as prednisolone.

These drugs are administered 'by the clock' and 'by the ladder'. In other words, one starts with the non-opioid drugs and adds adjuvant drugs if indicated. One then ascends the ladder to the weak opioids, which may be given either alone or in combination with non-opioids and adjuvants. If pain persists, strong opioids with or without non-opioids or adjuvants, are given. It is important that at each stage the patient and his pain are reassessed. Nurses and doctors should also consult the *British National Formulary*, updated each year, for information on side effects associated with the above-mentioned drugs.

COMBINATION OF PAIN RELIEF MEASURES

In the case of non-malignant pain, it is important to use drugs in combination with other relief measures and sometimes in combination with other drugs. Sometimes antidepressants and phenothiazines may help to relieve chronic pain. Amitriptyline can be useful, for example, in reducing the severity and frequency of migraine.

The goal of pain management in chronic pain is to try several strategies because the nature of chronic pain is complicated. Although analgesics are one line of therapy their prescription should be combined with offering the patient psychological input to help him or her to cope. Other chapters in this book have referred in some detail to the management of chronic pain.

TRANSCUTANEOUS ELECTRIC NERVE STIMULATION (TENS)

TENS can be used for the relief of both acute and chronic pain. The mechanism by which TENS results in pain relief is not understood, although there have been a number of suggested explanations. Some people feel that TENS activates nerve endings in the same way as the application of heat or cold. One possibility is that stimulating large diameter nerve fibres closes the gate (see Chapter 7) to the transmission of pain impulses (Nathan and Wall, 1974). Other suggestions are that TENS acts by blocking primary afferent nerve fibres or by stimulating the production of endorphins, the body's own naturally occurring opiate-like substances. For a really comprehensive overview of TENS (and other cutaneous methods of relieving pain), the reader is referred to McCaffery and Beebe (1994).

There are many kinds of electrical devices for TENS. These include small models, designed for patients to use themselves, which have a clip so they can be attached to a belt or put in a pocket. A TENS system basically consists of a battery-powered electronic pulse generator to which are connected 2–4 lead wires ending in electrodes that are placed on the skin.

Nurses should be acquainted with the use of TENS because they are ideally placed both in hospital and community settings to help and advise patients regarding its use. Patients with chronic pain often find a TENS machine helpful, sometimes in conjunction with other therapies. The machine should be positioned so that the patient finds it easy to adjust the controls.

The positioning of the electrodes is important. They are usually placed over the area of a peripheral nerve innervating the painful site. The best place may be nearest to the pain, but sometimes the patient may find relief when the electrodes are placed away from the painful site. Different patients report different effects from the use of TENS. Some patients only find relief from pain during stimulation while others may report periods of relief following treatment. These differences may reflect the variations in the nature of their pain. Patients should therefore adjust the controls according to their own needs. The stimulation is felt by the patient as a tingling or buzzing sensation and this can be adjusted by the knobs on the side of the unit. The patient can adjust the sensation until it is pleasant and relieves the pain. Some electrodes need an application of conductive gel. Self-adhesive electrodes are now available and are becoming more popular. There are reusable as well as disposable ones. A patient can wear the unit for as long as he likes. The electrodes can be left in place and the leads reattached when necessary. Sometimes the skin may become irritated and changing the tape used to keep the electrodes in place may help. If a rash occurs from the gel, then another type of gel should be substituted.

TENS may be used to treat all types of chronic pain, but the results are variable. Some patients experience complete relief while others have none. TENS may also be used for relief of postoperative pain. Sterile, pre-gelled electrodes may be placed close to a wound and left in place. A stimulator can then be connected when required. Deep breathing, coughing, and moving may be facilitated by the use of a TENS unit, which may reduce the need for opioid analgesia. If a TENS unit is to be used postoperatively it is useful if the patient can be made familiar with it prior to surgery. TENS is also useful in labour pain.

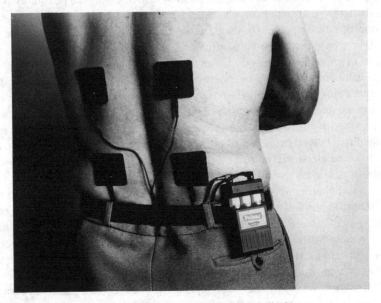

Figure 8.2 Application of TENS. (Courtesy of Spembly Medical.)

ACUPUNCTURE ANALGESIA

Acupuncture is a system of medicine developed by the ancient Chinese. During acupuncture treatment, fine needles pierce the skin at certain points on the body where particular effects can be obtained. The needles may be rotated or stimulated.

The Chinese explanation of how acupuncture analgesia works is based on the idea that life force flows around certain lines on the body known as meridians. Needling points on these lines is thought to correct an abnormal flow of life forces (Mann, 1971). Another explanation is that acupuncture stimulates the production of endorphins (Mayer, Price and Raffii, 1976).

Some acupuncturists use traditional Chinese acupuncture points which may not necessarily be near the site of pain. Others use trigger points, which are small, very sensitive regions in the muscle or connective tissue. They may be in the area of the pain or at some distance from it. Sometimes trigger points and acupuncture points correspond.

Pressure and massage on trigger points may relieve pain. Some therapists try using acupuncture points in this way, rather than needling the points. This is called acupressure. Illustrations of acupuncture points are shown in other (specialist) publications (Mann, 1971; McCaffery, 1983).

Acupuncture analgesia may be helpful in relieving some forms of chronic pain and has been found to be particularly useful in the treatment of migraine (Lipton, 1979) and chronic musculoskeletal pain. It is not effective in treating advanced cancer pain.

NERVE BLOCKS

In certain circumstances, perhaps when other methods of pain relief are con-traindicated or have proved ineffective, and where pain is unilateral and restricted to a particular area, a local nerve block may be considered. In this pro-cedure, the conduction of the nerve impulses which give rise to pain is prevented by injecting a local anaesthetic, which produces a temporary effect, or a drug that destroys the nerve fibres (neurolytic agent), such as phenol, producing a longer term effect.

Nerve blocks are carried out by doctors, usually anaesthetists, but the nurse should play a supportive role before and during the procedure and should also be aware of possible complications, some of which are specific to different types of nerve block. For example, following epidural anaesthesia there may be uri-nary retention. After any phenol injection, the exact position of the patient, as specified by the doctor, is crucial and should be maintained for one hour. In addition, observation of the patient for signs of hypotension and haematoma is obligatory for two hours after the procedure. Local anaesthetic blocks may be effective for up to 12–18 hours, whereas a phenol block may be effective for 8–22 weeks. The use of nerve blocks for the relief of chronic pain is discussed extensively by Latham (1983).

OTHER INVASIVE PROCEDURES

There are a number of other invasive techniques used by pain management doc-tors to try and relieve chronic pain. These include radiofrequency, cryotherapy and chemical neurolysis. These procedures are usually carried out in an operating theatre on patients who are day cases.

Acknowledgement

I am grateful to Dr J. Stock, Consultant Anaesthetist, and Mrs S. Whiteway, Lead Nurse Theatres, for permission to reproduce a synopsis of protocols used at the Conquest Hospital, Hastings.

References

British National Formulary No. 33 (1997) British Medical Association and Royal Pharmaceutical Society of Great Britain, London.

Carter, B. (1994) *Child and Infant Pain*, Chapman and Hall, London.

Copp, L. (1974) The spectrum of suffering. *American Journal of Nursing*, **74**(3), 491–5.

Egan, K. J. and Ready, B. (1994) Patient satisfaction with intravenous PCA or epidural morphine. *Canadian Journal of Anaesthesia*, **4**(11), 6–11.

Grant, S. (1997) Staff perceptions of pain management in accident and emergency departments. Unpublished BSc dissertation, University of Brighton.

Jaffe, J. H. (1975) Drug addiction and drug abuse, in *The Pharmacological Basis of Therapeutics*, 5th edn, (eds L. S. Goodman and M. Gilman), Macmillan, Basingstoke, pp. 284–324.

Johnson, D. and Spielberger, C. (1968) The effects of relaxation training and the passage of time on measures of state and trait anxiety. *Journal of Clinical Psychology*, **24**, 20.

Keeri-Szanto, M. and Heaman, S. (1972) Postoperative demand analgesia. *Surgery, Gynaecology and Obstetrics*, **134**, 646–51.

Latham, J. (1983) 1. The pain relief team. *Nursing Times*, (27 April), 54–7. 2. The nervous system. *Nursing Times*, (4 May), 56–60. 3. Complications. *Nursing Times*, (11 May), 36–8. 4. The nurse's role. *Nursing Times*, (18 May), 33–5.

Latham, J. (1990) *Pain Control*. Austen Cornish Ltd with The Lisa Sainsbury Foundation, London.

Lipton, S. (1979) Treatment of chronic pain, in *The Control of Chronic Pain*, (ed. S. Lipton), Edward Arnold, London.

Lynch, E. P., Lazor, M. A., Gellis, J. E. *et al.* (1997) Patient experience of pain after elective noncardiac surgery. *Anaesthesia and Analgesia*, **85**, 117–23.

Mann, F. (ed.) (1971) *Acupuncture: The Ancient Chinese Art of Healing*, Heinemann, London.

Mayer, D. J., Price, D. D. and Raffii, A. (1976) Antagonism of acupuncture analgesia in man by the narcotic antagonist naloxone. *Brain Research*, **121**, 36–7.

McCaffery, M. (1983) *Nursing the Patient in Pain*, Harper and Row, London.

McCaffery, M. and Beebe, A. (1994) *Pain. Clinical Manual for Nursing Practice*, (UK ed. J. Latham), Mosby, London.

Melzack, R. and Wall, P. D. (1996) *The Challenge of Pain*, Penguin Books, London.

Nathan, P. W, and Wall, P. D. (1974) Treatment of postherpetic neuralgia by prolonged electric stimulation. *British Medical Journal*, **3**, 645–7.

Payne, S. and Walker, J. (1996) *Psychology for Nurses and the Caring Professions*, Open University Press, Buckingham.

Sandler, A. N. (1994) Post-operative analgesia and patient satisfaction. *Canadian Journal of Anaesthesia*, **41**(1), 1–2.

Selbst, M. and Clark, M. (1990) Analgesic use in the Emergency Department. *Annals of Emergency Medicine*, **19**(9), 99–102.

Sofaer, B. (1984) The effect of focused education for nursing teams on postoperative pain of patients. Unpublished PhD thesis, University of Edinburgh.

Tamsen, A., Hartvig, P., Fagerlund, C., Dahlstrom, B. and Bondesson, U. (1982) Patient controlled analgesic therapy: clinical experience, *Acta Anaesthesiologica Scandinavica*, **74** (Suppl), 156–60.

Twycross, R. G. (1994) *Pain Relief in Far Advanced Cancer*, Churchill Livingstone, Edinburgh.

Vickers. M. (1985) Clinical trials of analgesic drugs, in *Patient Controlled Analgesia*, (eds M. Harmer, M. Rosen and M. Vickers), Blackwell Scientific, London.

Weiner, C. L. (1975) Pain assessment on an orthopaedic ward. *Nursing Outlook*, **23**, 506–16.

<table>
<tr><td>9</td><td># Feelings about pain and sympathetic listening</td></tr>
</table>

I wish no living thing to suffer pain.

Prometheus Unbound
Shelley

Let humanity ever be our goal.

Goethe

In this final chapter the feelings of patients and health professionals are discussed and some ways of lending a sympathetic ear are suggested.

FEELINGS OF PATIENTS

When people feel pain they experience a wide range of feelings and express them in a variety of ways. One man had an attack of renal colic and afterwards he said, 'You feel feeble saying so, but it is appallingly debilitating'. Another man, who had experienced years of increasing pain due to osteoporosis, said, 'I used to love all people, but in the past six months or so I have begun to dislike the human race. I get cross with my family, my friends and my colleagues. It is anger due to the pain really'. So people do recognize when pain has an effect on their emotions and their lives. But it is one thing to suffer and have relief, it is quite something else to be refused relief or to have to wait for it.

Negative feelings related to unrelieved acute pain may impede a patient's recovery and delay rehabilitation. In addition, patients may view the prospect of any future hospitalization with anxiety and trepidation. For example, one patient said that if she had to go into hospital again, 'I would be awfully anxious, extremely anxious and, I mean, I really couldn't go through taking that pain again. It was terrible. I just wouldn't go in again if I knew something similar was to happen to me'. Later, when asked if, despite her extreme anxiety, she felt that she would have a little more courage to ask for information for herself, she replied, 'Yes, I think I would. I don't think I would sort of freeze up when everybody comes round the bed and looks at you. I think I would be able to ask exactly what was happening and what they were doing rather than just leave it and not have them tell me a thing'.

On the other hand patients who have had good pain control really appreciate the efforts of nurses and doctors. One patient said:

I felt so awful really, complaining, but the nurse said I mustn't blame myself, that sometimes a drug works for one person and not another. She phoned the doctor and he came to the ward to see me. Then a few minutes later she came and gave me an injection. I'm not fond of injections, but it really helped and I was able to sleep. The next day I felt fine and so I was able to go home.

Patients suffering chronic pain are in a different position, but they may also be affected by initial inadequate treatment, although the situation may be more tolerable if at least those around these patients are interested in them as people. So often patients suffering chronic pain are referred back and forth from specialist to specialist. A number may be referred to a pain relief clinic, where they will find an interested doctor and/or nurse and, depending on the local organization, perhaps a multidisciplinary team.

Most patients who have suffered pain appreciate an outlet for expression of their feelings, whether they are being cared for at home, in a hospital ward or as an outpatient. The needs of patients vary according to the characteristics of their pain. Patients who have experienced unrelieved acute pain may feel that ventilation of feelings on one or a few occasions may spur them along the road to recovery. Patients experiencing unrelieved chronic benign pain may require frequent sessions to help them to come to terms with living with pain and to guide them towards an increased quality of life. For patients who have the pain of malignant disease there is the deepest suffering – what Cecily Saunders (1978) has called 'total pain' – a combination of physical, emotional, social and spiritual suffering.

The feelings patients experience when pain is not relieved vary with personality, previous pain experiences, expectations of health professionals and available therapies. It is important for health carers to realize that patients often need help to express these feelings and that they may experience great relief simply on being made to feel free to do this. However, health professionals should not 'force the issue' but facilitate natural expressions of feelings. One patient after discharge from hospital said, 'I am resentful against the hospital because they [the staff] should have warned you about how to cope and about what was going to happen and what you were going to go through. There wasn't the opportunity to talk about it'.

Working through feelings with patients

Sometimes it helps a person to talk about the meaning he attaches to pain. An open discussion of issues and problems will highlight areas for discussion. The goals of any discussion should include physical and psychological interventions. A person suffering chronic pain needs to assume some responsibility for treatment and may need to relearn how to live in the present rather than constantly referring back to the past (discussed in Chapter 2).

In order for the patient to function in the present, it is necessary to identify which feelings are causing the most problems so that they can be enabled to deal with them. For example, for some people frustration or fear prevents them from functioning normally. When they manage to discuss these feelings and find they are accepted and believed, they frequently develop insight and stop being over-burdened by them. For the most part one should work towards achieving a realistic balance. This means confronting issues such as utilization of time, consideration of others (i.e. family, friends and health professionals) and disowning bad habits.

Working with people who suffer chronic pain requires time. Health professionals need patience because we also can feel frustrated by 'non-responders' to treatment. It helps to discuss problems and share feelings in a team.

When patients are seen in a specialist pain management unit they often express surprise at being listened to, being heard and finding trust. But these should be available to any patient from any health professional and patients shouldn't have to go from 'pillar to post' to find them.

One danger of seeing several specialists or of trying several therapies unsuccessfully is the possibility that patients become demanding and egocentric. Sometimes patients spend time and money trying different treatments and become progressively dispirited. One lady said:

I had terrible pain in my face so I went to my GP. He sent me to a dentist who took out my teeth but that made the pain worse so I saw a maxillofacial surgeon. He could do nothing for me so I went to an osteopath. That was a waste of money so I tried reflexology. That was two years ago. That didn't work but my neighbour told me about Chinese medicine. The doctor there said he could cure me, but it didn't work so I tried acupuncture. I had 15 sessions but I felt no better. I feel miserable about life. I am angry and frustrated that nothing worked. I'll do anything to get rid of the pain.

Seeking help from inappropriate sources had repercussions for this patient but she did eventually seek help from a multidisciplinary team approach in a pain management unit.

Bridging the gap between fear and confidence, isolation and belonging, bad habits and good habits, poor time management and good time management are all tasks which a chronic pain patient should be prepared to take responsibility for and needs help with. I find that talking about these issues will highlight for different patients where they are finding 'blocks'. One patient expressed her isolation as follows: 'I feel isolated and alone. We used to have a lot of friends. They don't come to see us any more'.

Aftermath of pain

When pain is relieved or brought under control, patients sometimes still appreciate the opportunity to express feelings about the effects of pain when it is not controlled. When the cause of pain is removed, the patient needs to be told. For example, following a painful procedure such as a sterno-marrow puncture, patients might find it easier to relax once they know what is happening. On the other hand, a patient should not be told that a procedure is over and that there is no possibility of further discomfort until this is so, since a second attempt at the procedure may be required.

Some patients need to know that their behaviour while in pain was acceptable and normal. A feeling of having lost control may lessen a person's self-esteem. One patient said, 'I felt I had to apologize to the nursing staff for my behaviour but I was in such agony'. (In this particular case the analgesia provided had been inadequate.) Sometimes it helps patients to know that other people react in a similar way. Efforts to raise self-esteem following painful experiences may be very worthwhile in preventing lingering anxiety and emotional feelings. One patient was heard by all the patients on a ward screaming while a very painful dressing was being done. The nurse was heard to say, 'I am sorry, I have to do this, I'll give you some pethidine in a minute'. What she should have done was to administer the analgesia before commencing the dressing. The patient felt it necessary to apologize to all the other patients for 'making a noise'. This was a particularly unnecessary and ridiculous situation, which was distressing to many people and totally avoidable.

When pain is only partially controlled, some patients may feel relieved and express this, whereas others may experience feelings of fatigue from accumulated pain. Some prefer to forget about the pain and try to put it at the back of their minds. Others do not forget so easily and encouragement to express feelings may help.

When patients who have suffered chronic pain recognize that improvement has occurred, they may have problems adjusting to their former activities. One patient was able to resume doing a little gardening when pain in his leg improved but the enjoyment was hard for him to regain because he was afraid the pain would recur. In helping such a patient, it is useful to remember that social, physical and financial changes may have occurred during the time he suffered. Added to this are possible personality changes brought about by despair and depression. Prolonged pain may leave a person feeling isolated and angry with the world. Rehabilitation may require assistance and understanding from the nurse so that the patient can regain former confidence and increase his appreciation of life. Life may never be as it was formerly; efforts to help the patient to express feelings about this may aid progress towards new ways of fulfilment.

FEELINGS OF NURSING STAFF

Nursing provides the opportunity to develop nurturing skills, but for many the job is a stressful one. Many nurses develop feelings of powerlessness and frustration when they are unable to relieve suffering and may blame themselves or others. Unfortunately, when a nurse does become stressed (for this reason or any of a number of other reasons that make the job a stressful one), there may be a tendency for colleagues to assume that she cannot cope.

It has been pointed out (Latimer, 1980) that it is difficult being involved so closely on a day-to-day basis with other people's suffering. One student nurse wrote about the experience of working on a ward where all the staff had been involved in a programme about pain management. She said, 'It was rewarding to be involved in a team where there was open discussion about individual patients' pain relief'. She later contrasted this with a ward where she subsequently worked and felt frustrated at the lack of awareness among members of staff.

A student who had attended several lectures on the nursing management of pain subsequently went to work in an A&E department and was distressed by the following incident. A man arrived with chest pain, a possible myocardial infarction. On his arrival the care area was very busy; his initial recordings were carried out but he had to wait about 1½ hours before any decision was made as to what ward he should go to. Meanwhile, his relatives were waiting round the corner in a waiting area, obviously very worried about his condition. The patient was ashen-white, sweating and obviously in a considerable amount of distress.

Another student nurse was very unhappy about a certain event when on night duty. A third-year nurse was on night duty with her at the time. The student nurse commented:

> A patient returned from theatre and was suffering great physical and psychological pain. He was given an injection of diamorphine but this obviously was not adequate or appropriate for this man's pain. The third-year nurse informed the night sister when she came around. Sister told us to wait half an hour and if the patient's condition had not improved to inform the doctor. Meanwhile the patient's pain was not relieved.

Birch (1979) has also noted that failure to relieve pain is one cause of stress in student nurses. In order not to face the discomfort that a patient's suffering evokes, nurses may avoid a patient. This is an attempt to shut off the reality of the failure and guilt on the part of the nurse. Accumulation of these feelings of frustration and powerlessness may lead to depression and, in some cases, great unhappiness. Nurses may even leave nursing due to lack of job satisfaction.

For a patient, prolonged pain is demoralizing and frightening. If carers avoid patients, they may become withdrawn and preoccupied with pain. It is important that the nurse spends time with a patient and acknowledges the reality of a person's pain. Indicating that she is willing to stay with a patient and share facing the pain will be of great support and comfort to a patient. This is one constructive way of handling the feelings aroused in a nurse when she cares for a patient whose pain she cannot alleviate.

In the care of the terminally ill patient, a nurse may fear being the one who administers the last dose of analgesic before death. This can be particularly distressing if it has been necessary to increase the dose of opioid to control the pain, since the nurse may feel that she is in some way responsible for the patient's death. This distress is understandable and colleagues should be supportive of each other in such situations.

Nurses' stress may also be relieved by more open discussion of feelings in the ward situation. Nurse teachers should encourage learners to approach trained staff in a constructive way about issues that are concerning them and trained staff should be encouraged to acquire the skills necessary to deal sensitively with such situations. Another aspect of the problem is the task of raising awareness in all levels of staff regarding the importance of pain management in general. This is an area for discussion within continuing education and must be given priority.

Sometimes nurses who have had a lot of clinical experience find it difficult to change attitudes to managing pain despite recent research findings which clearly set out the benefits for patients. Whether or not to believe patients seems to be a recurring issue. Over a decade ago Sofaer (1984) found that 75% of nurses working in surgical wards reported that patients sometimes exaggerated pain. In a small study which included replication of a question relating to exaggeration of pain, Grant (1997) found exactly the same response in nurses working in accident and emergency departments.

ONE WAY OF LEARNING ABOUT FEELINGS

Sometimes it may be difficult for health professionals to understand the feelings of patients who experience pain and to understand their own feelings in relation to providing pain relief. The following exercise in role play is one which was tried out in a research project that initially led to writing this book. The participants were nurses who worked in surgical wards, but it has been used in classroom situations as well and in settings with medical students. Students could initiate this role play themselves. Alternatively, a teacher might like to use the idea.

Role play is a valuable aid to learning and one way in which learners may be encouraged to explore their attitudes to pain. However, its use should always be supervised, in the first instance at least, by experienced teachers. Care should also be taken that participants adopt pseudonyms and students are de-roled at the conclusion. A minimum of six people in the group is recommended, with no limitations on the maximum number, as those not actually role playing act as observers. The exercise is in two parts with two separate themes. The players are each briefed in private.

Part 1

A participant is asked to act out the role of a patient in severe pain. The other player is given the role of a disbelieving, busy nurse. The players are allowed to act the situation, until it spontaneously concludes (average time five minutes). Following the conclusion of the role play, each player is asked to relate her feelings in the role. These are noted on a blackboard if one is available. Finally, each player is de-roled by saying who she is in real life and not the role she played. Observers are requested not to discuss their observations among themselves. Part 2 of the exercise is then started.

Part 2

Two participants are again required and each is briefed privately. One person is asked to act the role of a patient in severe pain and the other of a nurse who believes the patient. The role play continues until it concludes spontaneously (average time two minutes). Each role player is asked how she feels and the comments are recorded as before. Participants are then de-roled. Following the role play, observers are asked for their comments on the nature of these interactions and a comparison is made.

Try out the above exercise and then compare your emerging themes with ours (Figure 9.1). (It has been found best to choose a particularly sympathetic nurse for the role of the disbeliever in Part 1. In this way the group can be supportive of her later, knowing that she would never behave like that in real life.)

	Theme 1	*Theme 2*
Some points usually noted by observers Length of time of interactions	Long	Short
Tone of voices used	High pitched and fast	Calm
Non-verbal clues	No touching	Touching
	No eye-to-eye contact	Eye-to-eye contact
	Nurse above patient	Same level
Feelings of nurse	Anger	Sympathy
	Insecurity	Autonomy
Feelings of patient	Anger	Empathy
	Frustration	Involvement
	Powerlessness	

Figure 9.1 Role play.

This exercise may sound simple, but it has been valuable in its simplicity because it demonstrates very clearly to nurses the implications of patient–nurse interactions. It is thought provoking to consider the effects that nurses themselves can create in a learning situation using role play. Reports from teacher colleagues who have used this exercise indicate that it is effective.

Several nurses have said of this exercise, 'It makes you think'. As Bond (1979) has stated:

> Where nurses have been taught to understand patients' pain and to deal with it by physical and psychological means, patients express a much greater degree of satisfaction with treatment than where the staff have not received any training of this kind.

DESPITE SCIENTIFIC ADVANCES, PEOPLE STILL SUFFER PAIN

Much progress has been made in recent years in techniques to relieve pain. Many words have been spoken and many articles and books have been published. But people still suffer pain. Even when many techniques have been tried, patients often return to pain clinics and report they still have pain. Even after wise people have spoken at conferences and published in reputable journals, people still suffer pain.

What may be difficult for students of pain to understand, is why so many scientists, therapists, physicians and others who acknowledge pain and its expression as a subjective phenomenon, sometimes tend to forget that each individual who experiences pain also has a unique set of life experiences that go hand in hand with the pain. These events and experiences, past and present, need to be explored in the context of the pain, alongside therapeutic interventions, if and when appropriate.

Pain cannot be set apart from other events in life. Acute pain may have a foreseeable end, but its interpretation and meaning for a patient is in the context of his own framework and not of ours. The person who suffers chronic pain will see his pain in the context of his life events, past, present and possibly future. The person who is at the end of life and in pain will be searching for peace of mind, along with pain relief.

As far as health professionals are concerned, most nurses intuitively realize these facts and are well placed to help assess and assist all pain sufferers. What is required is the confidence and skills to implement support for patients, knowledge regarding the wide range of techniques and therapies that exist and the ability to communicate effectively with other health professionals for the benefit of patients. Arthur Kleinman (1988), in his book *The Illness Narratives*, comments that in case conferences where multidisciplinary teams were discussing the pain of patients, 'the nurses, physiotherapists, occupational therapists and social worker often had more important information to contribute than did the medical specialist, but they clearly occupied a lower status and were overruled by the pain experts.'

This introductory book is intended to encourage nurses and other health professionals to further their thoughts and ideas on how best to help people who suffer pain. It is worth pointing out that no textbook can provide the experience to cope either with pain itself or with the pain of others and that so-called 'physical pain' is not an entity removed from psychological anguish, although people express it and cope with it in diverse ways.

Pain is a complex phenomenon experienced in the context of the complexity of human nature. Chronic pain particularly throws that normal complexity further into chaos and may produce crisis situations for the sufferer. Pain clinics, developed to try and sort out 'the problems', operate in different ways, some being staffed by a variety of specialists ranging from consultant anaesthetists and a team of psychologists to other specialists providing a range of therapies operating at a less sophisticated level.

PAIN: 'A CULTURE'

What is important, no matter where pain is being treated, is one's attitude to and understanding of patients. Finer (1991) utilizes the concept of 'a pain culture' – the values that patients and health professionals expressed to each other by virtue of the worlds they live in. The patient lives in a world of pain and the language he uses to express his living is derived from that world. The doctors and nurses, on the other hand, are well and not 'in pain'. (Although they may well suffer the 'anguish' of failure to help others.) Somehow or other, for empathy and understanding to develop, both patient and health carer have to understand the world of the other. Pain therapy therefore has to be based on shared responsibility between patient and therapist. What complicates the issue further is that often several therapies may be tried out and so communication and understanding have to develop between the health carers themselves. This takes time, requires an understanding of each other's qualities, attributes and skills and, in order to be of benefit to patients, has to be well co-ordinated. This applies in both acute and chronic settings.

NURSES AND NURSING

Many nurses are experienced 'therapists' without realizing it and others need help with education to boost confidence in developing skills. What is beginning to happen in nursing is the realization, with theoretical backing (though to some people it has always been common sense), that a human being goes through different stages of life and development, is subject to ups and downs and has a role in controlling his own life. This realization is *crucial* to the management of pain, for it is the control of the balance between pain and pleasant feelings that makes life livable and bearable for some and the lack of control that makes life and living intolerable and unbearable for others. For those who have lost control, helping them to restore the balance may involve the acceptance by people who suffer chronic pain that pain and pleasant feelings may coexist. In other words, 'living with the pain' – a phrase much used and abused, misunderstood and brandished about, should be interpreted as meaning living a life that involves positive feelings about oneself and the world, as well as having the pain. This is difficult for many people to accept; they want the pain doctor and the nurse to 'take it away'. Nurses can develop a therapeutic relationship such that patients are able to accept help. The first stage is nurses' acceptance of the expression of pain by the patient. Lip service is often paid to 'patient individuality'. It would be better to take individuality for granted rather than to talk about it!

COUNSELLING

Counselling is a useful approach which may be used by nurses and other health professionals in many health-care settings. It is one way of providing confidential psychological help to people who suffer pain, particularly chronic pain. It can be practised at different levels and there is a wide choice in the way one can learn to become a counsellor. However, it is wise to seek advice from the British Association of Counselling before undertaking a counselling course in order to ensure that a particular course meets their criteria for accreditation.

One approach, particularly suited to use with chronic pain patients, is known as 'person centred counselling'. It was developed by Dr Carl Rogers in the 1930s and 1940s and is non-directive. For further reading and examples of how counselling may be used in the management of chronic pain, see Sofaer (1998).

Experience with patients in a pain clinic

The following are two descriptions of work with patients in pain clinics and illustrate the kinds of things patients say they feel.

Mrs Q is a 57-year-old woman who has suffered back pain for many years. She says that she feels 'isolated'. Her husband has recently taken early retirement to 'look after her'. Her typical day begins at 7.30 am when she has a cup of tea brought to her in bed. She then gets up and after getting dressed, lies down again because she 'feels too weak with the exhaustion of having got dressed'. After a while she potters about the house. After lunch she lies down again. She has been married for 38 years, but it is a 'long time since lovemaking has taken place'. She has not been to a shop 'for several years'. She does her shopping by catalogue. She had a friend who used to visit her, but no longer feels she has any friends. She says it is several years since she has gone out except to the hospital, which takes several days of preparation. 'I admit', she says, 'that the pain has taken over my life; it is bigger in my mind than it need be'.

Mrs Q was encouraged to go for little walks, starting with three minutes and building up to one hour over a period of a month. She was encouraged to think about the areas of her life she would like to improve and especially to give thought to her personal and social situation. She agreed to setting some short-term goals to increase her quality of life. She started by taking short walks and then (because she found she really could do it), she developed a tendency to overdo the activity and required further advice, encouragement and counselling.

Mr P is in his late 70s. He was active in the Second World War. He lives with his wife and they have a harmonious and warm relationship. They cry together sometimes with frustration about the pain. He experiences back pain and is unable to walk for long periods or to sit at the table and eat in comfort and feels quite unable to participate in any social life. When asked what he would like to talk about, Mr P reminisced; when asked what he felt was shaping and colouring his life situation at the present time, he talked in great detail about the death and funeral of a relative many years ago. After some 40 minutes of reminiscing, he finally said, 'I know I am digging my own grave'. In consultation with his wife, it was decided that Mr P would begin to take note of the positive things in his life and with her help, they would recall the good times together. Mr and Mrs P drew up a list of distractions to help Mr P focus on more positive aspects of his life. He did this and things improved greatly for them both.

Over the years while practising as a counsellor I have met many people who suffer chronic pain. A particular problem for them seems to be being misunderstood and misperceived. Many seem to have poor relationships with family and friends and have developed a pattern of behaviour which often includes sleeping poorly and eating too much. (One patient ate ten bars of chocolate every morning yet he knew he was overweight and this was not helping his back problem!)

Helping to build a bridge

It may be useful to take your cue from the patient. Start where the patient starts. In my experience patients sometimes start to talk at the point where they want to express 'isolation' and 'fear'. If a patient can be allowed to express this he may show strong emotions with present or past experiences associated with a feeling of being unable to build a bridge for himself to enhance the quality of life and living. In order to help build that bridge, the health professional should guard against preconceived ideas, as so often medical colleagues and others refer to patients with pain as having 'emotional overlay'. This is due to a lack of acceptance by some health professionals that emotionality is naturally associated with the pain experience, an idea that people outside the world of nursing and medicine seem to have no difficulty with.

Inexperience

A major problem is when inexperienced carers find themselves dealing with complicated and difficult emotional problems. Of course, there is a wide variation in how people express feelings and not everyone wants or feels it appropriate to 'let it all hang out' with a stranger. This must be respected. However, generally speaking, people who suffer chronic pain often appreciate a sympathetic ear, which may be the first step for the patient in trying to recreate a positive image of himself and his world. If we are to be of real benefit to our patients who suffer pain, then it is essential to develop ways of assessing individual emotional responses and to assist patients subsequently in developing coping strategies. In this sort of situation you don't have to be a trained counsellor, but you may use counselling skills to try and understand and help the patient.

Do not underestimate your own first step, either. We will all learn by experience. Sometimes patients like to talk about the past and what they used to be able to do. (One young woman patient with multiple injuries following a road traffic accident talked endlessly about her past, particularly her sports activities, and it took several sessions before she would concentrate on the present or even give a thought to the future.) The kinds of feelings expressed often include sadness, despair, anger and grief. People in chronic pain have lost so much that the feelings of loss are sometimes overwhelming. One young man who had a serious accident which left him with chronic back pain said, 'I have lost my health and my ability to function, my girl friend left me and my mother died and now I have lost the business'.

Loneliness and isolation, especially if a person lives alone, may compound the difficulties. But these may be present too in a person who does not live alone, but feels isolated because of pain. One patient expressed this feeling as being the most difficult to cope with because she felt trapped in a marriage of 38 years with a husband who 'humiliated' her because he did not believe her pain.

One is often faced with the problem of how to 'enter the world' of another person's pain. The one thing that applies to all situations is that you should try to make good contact with the patient.

What does it feel like? Pain and more pain.
Darkness and silence and pain. Constant pain.
And no one can reach me ... no one has the sympathy,
the wisdom, the courage, to find their way inside.

My wilderness of pain.

To find the right words.
Or maybe you, for you've helped me speak.

David, Jerusalem, 1984

Sometimes nurses ask how it is possible to enter the world of another's pain and remain uninvolved emotionally. A non-nursing colleague asked if nurses are taught to 'remain professional' (meaning distant). 'If only they would come closer to her,' (referring to his elderly infirm mother), 'If only they would touch her, if only they would hold her hand.' He was reassured to hear that nurses are encouraged to touch, and to hold a hand as part of being a professional nurse.

People express their feelings in different ways. One should be guided by the sufferer. Many health professionals, particularly nurses, may find it easier to hold someone who is distraught and to cry with a person in consolation than to deal with angry feelings. It is important to remember that there is no right way to say anything and that if you are 'stuck' and do not know what to say, then be honest and say so. It is difficult to help people who suffer chronic pain, but don't give up! The following ideas may help.

- Make it clear that you hear what they are telling you. If it is not clear what the problem is, then clarify it.
- Make clear the time you have available to listen and give undivided attention. Don't get distracted by other things. If you can't listen now, don't promise 'to come back' if it is unlikely that you will be able to.
- Recall with the patient what was last said so that the patient knows you have heard.
- Don't make false promises. Pain is real. Maybe a technique will work. Maybe it won't.
- There is power in non-verbal communication. Socrates wrote about it:

Nobility and dignity, self-abasement and servility, prudence and understanding, insolence and vulgarity, are all reflected in the face and in the attitudes of the body whether still or in motion.

This applies to us all, to health professionals and to patients.

CONCLUDING THOUGHTS

This book has addressed the issues of the relationship between psychological factors and pain, cultural dimensions of pain expression, accountability and responsibility of health professionals (particularly nurses), communication between health professionals and patients and has introduced the reader to the science of pain and to some pain therapies. Vignettes and quotations from the lives of patients have also been used to illustrate some problems in pain management. New areas not addressed in this book are constantly being investigated in the world of pain research and therapies. The pain syndromes that affect patients who have AIDS and the problems faced by people with learning difficulties are just two issues which are beginning to receive attention.

The late Professor Eugene (John) Heimler was a man who spent most of his life helping others to cross the bridge from an unhappy and painful past to a positive present and hope for the future. His words about pain encapsulate what much of this book is about:

Do not ask 'why' pain, only what has to be done with it. *The Storm* (John Heimler)

In this book, the narratives of patients have been used to provide insights into their feelings. It isn't so easy to find examples of good practice, but then, probably good practice is less frequently documented in the literature than poor practice. Alexander, Fawcett and Runciman (1994), however, documented one case history (no. 10.3), an account by a patient of her perception of experiences surrounding a total hip replacement, which is very heartening. The patient, recalling her experiences two months following surgery, discusses the preoperative and postoperative care: 'preoperative relief of anxiety and postoperative pain relief were superb'. She notes that the absence of pain as a result of surgery predominates in her mind so much now 'that everything else fades into insignificance'.

On that encouraging note, I wish you 'good luck'. I hope that this book will help you in your own efforts to bring comfort and relief of pain to patients.

References

Alexander, M. F., Fawcett, J. N. and Runciman, P. J. (1994) *Nursing Practice. Hospital and Home. The Adult*, Churchill Livingstone, Edinburgh.

Birch, I. (1979) The anxious learners. *Nursing Mirror*, **148**, 17–22.

Bond, M. J. (1979) The influence of learning and the environment on pain, in *Pain: Its Nature, Analysis and Treatment*, (ed. M. J. Bond), Churchill Livingstone, Edinburgh.

Finer, B. (1991) Personal communication.

Grant, S. (1997) Perceptions of doctors and nurses towards pain management in accident and emergency. Unpublished BSc dissertation, University of Brighton.

Heimler, E. (1976) *The Storm* (trans. A. Rudolf), Menard Press, London.

Kleinman, A. (1988) *The Illness Narratives*, Basic Books, New York.

Latimer, J. (1980) Stress and the student nurse. *Nursing*, **10**, 449–50.

Saunders, C. (1978) *The Management of Terminal Illness*, Edward Arnold, London.

Sofaer, B. (1984) The effect of focused education for nursing teams on postoperative pain of patients. Unpublished PhD thesis, University of Edinburgh.

Sofaer, B. (1998) Counselling in the management of chronic pain, in *Perspectives on Pain: Mapping the Territory*, (ed. B. Carter), Edward Arnold, London.

Glossary

Acute pain An episode of pain of sudden onset, short duration and foreseeable end

Adaptation The process by which a patient may gradually manage to endure pain and carry on despite it, perhaps without obvious outward signs of pain

Analogue scale (for determining pain scores) A scale on which the extremes of pain experience (no pain, pain as bad as it can be) are indicated. The patient places a mark on the scale to represent the level of pain at the time and the distance of this mark in standard units from the 'no pain' end of the scale is taken as the pain score

Body chart Simple outlines of the front and back views of the body on which the site of a patient's pain can be recorded

Chronic pain Pain lasting for six months or more

Deep pain Pain originating in the organs of the body. It is usually not as well localized as superficial pain and has an aching quality

Drug dependence

(a) *Psychological dependence* 'The intense craving and compulsive perpetuation of abuse to repeat the desired effect of a psychotropic drug' (World Health Organization 1969)

(b) *Physical dependence* 'An adaptive state which manifests itself by intense physical disturbances when administration of the drug is suspended or when its action is affected by the administration of a specific antagonist' (World Health Organization 1969). With continued use of morphine or heroin, physical dependence usually takes place within weeks of the first dose

Drug tolerance The need, with long-term drug therapy, to administer increasingly large doses to produce the same effect

Opioids Drugs derived from opium. These can be synthetic or naturally derived

Pain assessment chart A written record, usually over a period of hours or days, of the intensity and site of a patient's pain and the actions taken to control it

Pain autobiography An individual's collective previous experience of pain

Pain description chart A list of adjectives that could be used to describe the intensity and quality of pain, used as an aid in pain assessment

Pain profile A record (usually graphic) of a patient's pain scores, usually over a period of hours or days, used to assess the response to pain-relieving measures

Pain threshold The least stimulus intensity at which a person perceives pain

Pain tolerance The greatest stimulus intensity causing pain that a person is prepared to tolerate

Psychogenic pain Pain with no detectable physical cause in a patient with a history of expressing emotional problems in terms of pain

Referred pain Pain felt at a site other than that which has been stimulated

State anxiety Anxiety that may be present in a patient facing a potentially stressful event

Superficial pain Pain originating from the stimulation of the skin or mucous membranes. It may be described as bright, pricking or burning and is usually localized

Further reading

Barber, J. and Adrian, C. (eds) *Psychological Approaches to the Management of Pain*, Brunner Mazel, New York.

Carroll, D. and Bewsher, D. (1993) *Pain Management and Nursing Care*, Butterworth-Heinemann, Oxford.

Carter, B. (ed.) (1998) *Perspectives on Pain: Mapping the Territory*, Edward Arnold, London, Sydney, Auckland.

Fagerhaugh, S. Y. and Strauss, A. (1977) *Politics of Pain Management*, Addison-Wesley, New York.

Gibson, H. B. (ed.) (1994) *Psychology, Pain and Anaesthesia*, Chapman and Hall, London.

International Association for the Study of Pain Subcommittee on Taxonomy (1979) Pain terms: a list with definitions and notes on usage. *Pain*, **6**, 249–52.

International Council of Nurses (1973) *Code for Nurses: Ethical Concepts Applied to Nursing*, International Council of Nurses, Geneva.

Kotarba, J. A. (1983) *Chronic Pain. Its Social Dimensions*, Sage Publications, Beverly Hills.

Latham, J. (1990) *Pain Control*, Austen Cornish Ltd with The Lisa Sainsbury Foundation, London.

McCaffery, M. (1983) *Nursing the Patient in Pain*, Harper and Row, London.

McCaffery, M. and Beebe, A. (1994) *Pain. Clinical Manual for Nursing Practice*. (ed. J. Latham), Mosby, London.

McGrath, P. J. and Unruh, A. M. (1987) *Pain in Children and Adolescents, Vol. 1, Pain Research and Clinical Management*, Elsevier, Amsterdam.

Melzack, R. and Wall, P. D. (1996) *The Challenge of Pain*, Penguin Books, London.

Royal College of Surgeons of England and the College of Anaesthetists (1990) *Report of the Working Party on Pain After Surgery*, Royal College of Surgeons of England and the College of Anaesthetists, London.

Thomas, V. N. (ed.) (1997) *Pain. Its Nature and Management*, Baillière Tindall, London.

Twycross, R. G. (1994) *Pain Relief in Far Advanced Cancer*, Churchill Livingstone, Edinburgh.

Index

Page numbers printed in *italic* refer to figures; those in **bold** type to definitions in the glossary

Accident and Emergency treatment 101
Accountability for pain relief 44–5
Acts of Parliament 91
Acupressure 105
Acupuncture 104–5
Acute pain 17–18, **122**
  analgesics for 100–1
  nurses' problems in managing 23
Acute trauma 18
Adaptation 21, **122**
Addiction to opioids 101
Adjuvants 102
Aftermath of pain 111–12
Amino acids 80–1
Amitriptyline 99, 102
Analgesia
  balanced 101
  postoperative 101
  see also Patient-controlled analgesia
Analgesic ladder 99–100, 102
Analgesics 90–102
  assessing efficacy of 53
  compound preparations 95
  management of acute pain 100–1
  management of chronic pain 102
  potency *100*
  recording effects of 46–7
  timing of medication 3, 4, 7, 73
  see also Non-opioids; Opioids; *and*
    specific drugs and drug types
Analogue scales 59–62, **122**

Anger 29
  of patients 6, 7, 8–9, 71
Anticonvulsants 102
Antidepressants 102
Antiemetics 92
Anxiety 28–9, 31
  state anxiety 89, **123**
Anxiolytics 102
Art 12–13
Arts, influence of 11–13
Aspartate 80, 81
Aspav 95, *100*
Aspirin 79, 95, 98, *100*, 102
Assessment of pain 52–66
  analogue scales 59–62, **122**
  assessment charts 58, *60–1*, **122**
  body charts 59, 62–3, **122**
  in children 59
  chronic pain 62–3
  difficulties in 56–7
  elderly patients 54, *55*
  home assessment records 63
  individualized 57–63
  intervals between 62, 63
  misconceptions in 56–7
  nurses' role in 39–40
  pain cues 53
  poor practices in 53
  prerequisites for nurses 64
  self-assessment 58
Awareness of pain

after distraction 86
on part of nurse 57
Axon reflex 79
Axsain 99

Back pain 15, 21
Balanced analgesia 101
Behaviour of patients
'but' 20
expectations of 42–3
hysterical 30
immature 20, 110
obsessional 30
patterns of 19–21
responses to 42–3
Beliefs 27–8
incongruence within caring team 42
professionals' 39–40
Bible 12
Biopsychosocial approach 84
Body charts 59, 62–3, **122**
Body image, threat to 31
Brain, response to pain 78, 81–2
Breathing, in relaxation 89–90
British Association of Counselling 117
British National Formulary 91, 100, 102
Bupivacaine 96, 101
Buprenorphine 91, 94, *100*, 102

Calcitonin gene-related peptide (CGRP)
80–1
Cancer pain 22
WHO guidelines 102
Carbamazepine 99, 102
CGRP (calcitonin gene-related peptide)
80–1
Children
assessment of pain 59
distraction methods 86
use of imagery 88
Chronic pain 18–19, **122**
analgesics for 102
assessment 62–3
nurses' problems in managing 23
stages 19
Co-codamol *100*
Co-codaprin 95, *100*
Codeine *100*, 102

Codeine phosphate 93–4, 95
Co-dydramol 95, *100*
Colour, in distraction 88
Comfort measures 63
Communication 47–9
see also Information for patients
Constipation, as side-effect of opioids 92
Control
and coping 27, 35
locus of control, and PCA 96
Controlled drugs 91
Coping 29–30
and control 27, 35
Coping strategies 54, 85–6
active *v.* passive 29–30
nurses' knowledge of patient's 27–8, 35
variations in style 30
Coping Strategies Questionnaire 29–30
Co-proxamol 95, *100*
Corticosteroids 102
Cough 94
Counselling 117–20
Counterirritants 99
Cryotherapy 105
Cultural factors 33–4
Anglo-Saxon 33
crosscultural research 34

Deep pain 16, **122**
Defining pain 15–16
Dependence, *see* Drug dependence
Depression 28, 31, 111
in nurses 112
Descending inhibitory control 78, 80, *82*
Dextromoramide 94
Dextropropoxyphene 102
Dextropropoxyphene hydrochloride 95
DF118 93
Diamorphine 91, 93, 96, *100*, 101
Diazepam 102
Diclofenac sodium 99
Diflunisal 98
Dihydrocodeine *100*
Dihydrocodeine tartrate 93, 95
Discussion
multidisciplinary 115
with patients 110–11
Distraction 85–6

Doctor–nurse interactions 47–9
Doctors, reliance on nurses 42, 47
Documentation, *see* Records
Dolobid 98
Dorsal horn cells 80
Drug addiction, opioids 101
Drug dependence, psychological and
　　physical **122**
　opioids 21
Drug rounds, constraints on patients 57
Drugs, *see* Analgesics; Misuse of Drugs
　　Act; Misuse of Drugs Regulations;
　　and specific drugs and drug types
Drug tolerance **122**
　morphine 92

Education
　pain relief 44
　by role play 113–15
Elderly patients 54, *55*
Emergency treatment 101
Emla 99
Emotions 27–8
Endorphins 81
Enkephalins 81
Entonox 101
Epidural infusions 96–7, 101
Ethics of pain relief 13–14
Ethnic groups 33–4
Extroverts *v.* introverts 27

Fatigue 30
Feelings about pain
　learning about 113–15
　of nursing staff 112–13
　of patients 108–12
Feldene 99
Fentanyl 96, 100, 101
Fortral 94
Frustration 29

Gate control theory 56, 76–8, 82
Gender differences, in pain perception 34
Glutamate 80, 81
Greek texts 11, 13

Haloperidol 102
Health professionals

attitudes transforming patients' feelings
　6, 70, 72, 74
　believing patients 7, 14, 15, 113
　power of 5–6, 7–8, 71, 73
　shared responsibility 20–1, 116
　see also Nurses
Helplessness of patients 5, 71–3
Heroin 93
Home assessment records 63
Hospitalization
　patients' fears and anxieties 3, 5, 31,
　　108–9
　patients' personal experiences 1-10, 67-
　　75
Hyperalgesia 79, 81
Hysteria 30

Ibuprofen 98, 102
Imagery 85, 86–8
Individuality
　in coping styles 30
　of life events 115
　and nursing models 52
　in pain assessment 57–63
　in pain responses 54–6
　of patients 15, 26, 35–6, 40, 117
　in response to treatment 85
Information for patients 28, 28–9, 35, 49
　patients' experiences 2, 4, 6, 70–1
Infusion pumps 95–6
Inhibitory processes 78, 80, *82*
　see also Gate control theory
Injury, detection of, *see* Nociception
International Association for the Study of
　　Pain 13, 44
International Council of Nurses 13
Interneurones 77
Intramuscular injection 101
Introverts *v.* extroverts 27
Isolation 19, 111, 119

Judgements, nurses' personal 40–1
Justice 14

Ladder of analgesic drugs 99–100, 102
Laxatives, with opioids 92
Learned helplessness 28
Learning, effect of 32–3

Lewis, C.S. 12
Life events, pain in context of 115
Listening, to the patient 20, 110
Literary perspectives 11–13
'Living with the pain' 116
Locus of control, and PCA 96

McGill Pain Questionnaire 35, 63
Management of pain
  elderly patients in the community *55*
  nurses' problems in 22–3
  pain management programmes 21–2
  preventative 100
  see also Analgesia; Analgesics; Pain
    relief; *and specific drugs, drug types
    and therapies*
Marcain 96, 101
Medication, timing of 3, 4, 7, 73
Mefenamic acid 98
Meptazinol *100*
Methadone 94
N-Methyl-D-aspartate (NMDA) receptor
  81
Migraine 102
Mild pain, analgesics for *100*
Misuse of Drugs Act (1971) 91
Misuse of Drugs Regulations (1985) 91
Modelling 32–3
Models of nursing 52
Moderate pain, analgesics for *100*
Montaigne, M. de 13, 74, 75
Moods 27–8
Morphine 91, 92, *100*, 101, 102
  side-effects 92
Multidisciplinary approach
  to pain relief 14–15, 15–16, 115, 116
  to pain study 13

Naloxone 92, 94, 97–8
Narphen 94
Nefopam *100*
Nerve blocks 105
Nerve fibres, sensory 78–9
Neurokinin A 80
Neuroleptics 102
Neurolysis 105
Neuropeptides 79, 80–1
Neurotransmitters 81

NMDA (N-methyl-D-aspartate) receptor
  81
Nociception 76
  peripheral events in 78–9
Non-opioids 21, 98, 102
  v. opioids 91
Non-steroidal anti-inflammatory drugs
  (NSAIDs) 79, 98–9, 99, *100*, 102
Nurse–doctor interactions 47–9
Nurses
  believing patients 7, 113
  drug administration role 90–1
  feelings of 112–13
  pain relief role 46–7
  patient assessment role 39–40
  patient avoidance 112
  and patients' behaviour 42–3
  patients' perception of 3–7, 71–3, 74
  personal judgements 40–1
  problems faced by 22–3
  roles of, from patients' viewpoints 64
  reliance of doctors on 42, 47
  stress in 112–13
  as therapists 116–17
  see also Health professionals
Nursing models 52

Obsessional behaviour of patients 30
Omeprazole 95
Omnopon 93
Opiates 91–4
Opioids **122**
  addiction 101
  administration protocols 17
  dependence 21
  endogenous 81
  intravenous 95
  laxatives with 92
  v. non-opioids 91
  strong 102
  weak 102

Pain
  assessment, *see* Assessment of pain
  definitions 15–16
  management, *see* Management of pain
  meaning of 34
  personal experiences of 1–10, 67–75

protection role of 78
relief of, *see* Pain relief
a subjective experience 14, 15, 52, 58
types of 16–19
Pain assessment charts 58, *60–1*, **122**
Pain autobiography 32, 39–40, **122**
Pain clinics 116
  patients' perspectives of 8, 9
Pain cues 53
Pain culture 116
Pain description chart **122**
Pain profile 62, *62*, **122**
Pain relief
  barriers to innovation in 52–3
  but suffering continues 115–16
  combination of measures 102
  education 44
  ethical principles 13–14
  geared to hospital routine 57
  lack of action on 44–5
  multidisciplinary approach 14–15,
    15–16, 115, 116
  priority? 4
  public's expectations 17, 27
  see also Analgesia; Analgesics;
    Management of Pain; *and specific
    drugs, drug types and therapies*
Pain Society 22
Pain system *82*
Pain threshold 27, **122**
Pain tolerance 54, **122**
  levels 33–4
Palfium 94
Papaveretum 93, 95, *100*
Paracetamol 95, 99, *100*, 102
Partnership 20, 35, 45–6
Patient-controlled analgesia (PCA) 96, 97,
  101
Patients
  anger of 6, 7, 8–9, 71
  as arbiters of pain 14, 15, 58
  discussion with 110–11
  fear and anxieties of hospitalization 3, 5,
    31, 108–9
  feelings of 108–12
  helplessness of 5, 71–3
  individuality of 15, 26, 35–6, 40, 117
  as partners 20, 35, 45–6
  personal experiences 1–10, 67–75
  previous experiences of pain 31, 32
  reports of pain 56
  responses to pain 54–6
  self-assessment of pain 58
  self-esteem, loss of 111
  shared responsibility 20–1, 116
  views of 63–4
PCA, *see* Patient-controlled analgesia
Pentazocine 91, 94
Peptides 79, 80–1
Peripheral nervous system 76, *82*
Personality, patient's 27, 35
  changes 111–12
Personal judgements, professionals' 40–1
Person-centred counselling 117
Pethidine 91, 93, 96, *100*, 101, 102
Phantom limb pain 35–6
Phenazocine 94
Phenol 105
Phenothiazines 102
Physeptone 94
Physiology 78
Placebo response 16
Poetry 12
Ponstan 98
Postoperative analgesia 101
Postoperative pain 17, 71–3
Power
  v. accountability 44–5
  of health professionals 5–6, 7–8, 71, 73
Prednisolone 102
Prochlorperazine 92, 102
Professionals, *see* Health professionals
Psychiatric illnesses 31
Psychogenic pain 30–1, **123**
Psychological factors 26–32
  combination of 32
  implications for nursing 31–2
  sources of stress 31–2
Psychological support 35–6
Punishment, pain as 31, 34

Ranitidine 95
Records 46–7, 58, 62, 63
Referred pain 17, **123**
Regulations 91
Rehabilitation 111–12

Relaxation 88–90
Research, crosscultural 34
Respiratory depression 92, 93, 94, 97–8
Responses to pain 54–6
Responsibility, shared 20–1, 116
Role play 113–15
Routine, in hospitals 57

Schizophrenia 31
Self-assessment of pain 58
Self-esteem, patient's loss of 111
Sensitization 79
Sensory nerve fibres 78–9
Severe pain, analgesics for *100*
Shoes, back pain patients 21
Sickle cell disease 22
Solpadol *100*
Specialists' different perspectives 15
Spinal cord 76, 80–1, *82*
State anxiety 89, **123**
Stereotyping 35
Stress 89
    in nurses 112–13
Student nurses, stress in 112
Subjective nature of pain 14, 15, 52, 58
Substance P 79, 80, 81
Substantia gelatinosa 77, 80, 82
Superficial pain 16, **123**
Support, psychological 35–6
'Supratentorial' 30

Tegretol 99
Temgesic 94
TENS (transcutaneous electric nerve

stimulation) 103–4
Terminally-ill patients 23, 113
Therapies 84–107
    see also individual therapies
Thresholds, *see* Pain threshold
Tissue damage 56–7
Tolerance, *see* Drug tolerance; Pain
    tolerance
Topical preparations 99
Total pain 109
Tradition, *see* Routine
Training, *see* Education
Tramadol *100*
Transcutaneous electric nerve stimulation
    (TENS) 103–4
Trigger points 104–5
Trust 14, 19–20
Tylex *100*

Undertreatment 53, 101
Uniqueness, *see* Individuality

Values, professionals' 39–40
    incongruence within caring team 42
Vanderbilt Pain Management Inventory
    (VPMI) 29
Voltarol 99, *100*

Weather changes 21
WHO, *see* World Health Organization
'Wind up' process 77
World Health Organization (WHO),
    guidelines for relief of cancer pain
    102